About the author

Kate Mikhail is a London-based freelance journalist and editor, who has written a wide range of features and reviews for the *Guardian, Observer, Telegraph* and *Independent* newspapers, as well as for many other publications.

After decades of not being able to get to sleep easily at night, a chance reading of a book by her great-great-uncle Richard Waters, a pioneer in cognitive therapy and clinical hypnosis, led to the discovery that she was officially a chronic insomniac. A love of research, science and a fascination with the mind–body loop, drove Kate to find scientific answers for why sleep can be such a problem for so many people in the 21st century, and what can be done to put this right.

Kate is now an ex-chronic insomniac, thanks to researching *Teach Yourself to Sleep*, in which she explores the biology and science of sleep and how to look at sleep from a different perspective to improve the quality of sleep, health and wellbeing.

katemikhail.com

KATE MIKHAIL

Teach Yourself To Sleep

An ex-insomniac's guide

PIATKUS

PIATKUS

First published in Great Britain in 2021 by Piatkus

1 3 5 7 9 10 8 6 4 2

A CIP catalogue record for this book
is available from the British Library.

ISBN 978-0-349-42816-1

Typeset in Garamond by M Rules
Printed and bound in Great Britain by
Clays Ltd, Elcograf S.p.A

Papers used by Piatkus are from well-managed forests
and other responsible sources.

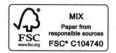

Piatkus
An imprint of
Little, Brown Book Group
Carmelite House
50 Victoria Embankment
London EC4Y 0DZ

An Hachette UK Company
www.hachette.co.uk

www.littlebrown.co.uk

For Chris

Contents

Why Bother Sleeping (Much) – and Where to Begin

Everything about our day feeds into our night, dictating the quality of our sleep, which controls the quality of tomorrow.

We used to sleep on the ground, sometimes on straw, and had all kinds of rituals at night to make sure that we were safe from thieves, fires, disease and demons, and that we were bug-free. So if our distant ancestors could see us now, snuggled down in our deluxe nests, they might well ask, 'Why *on earth* can't you sleep well?'

If only sleep was that simple, but for millions of us across the globe it isn't. The fear and discomfort of old have been replaced by the stress and over-stimulation of modern life, which can make it hard for us to switch off at night, or to stay asleep. The artificial light that surrounds us is disconnecting us from night and day and our natural sleep–wake cycle, and unwanted sleep patterns can quickly become habitual, tenacious and resistant to change.

Comfy bed or not, I could never take sleep for granted. My problem was that I couldn't always get to sleep that easily. Instead I would often lie awake half the night, my mind buzzing, increasingly wired and anxious, waiting for sleep to show up, and then be groggy in the morning when the alarm went off.

It can be less gruelling to wing life on too little sleep when you're younger, of course, especially if you don't have children, which I didn't in my twenties or for most of my thirties. Also, my life as a journalist was never a nine-to-five set-up, so it was flexible enough for me to get by. And although I can remember the knot in my stomach and the rising anxiety, the more strained with exhaustion I became at 2am or 3am, knowing that I had to get up for work just a few hours later, it was only occasionally very bad – besides, I had sleeping pills within reach as a last resort. Not that pills were any match for a good night's sleep, of course. They left me feeling leaden and metallic inside come morning, but having a few hours' sleep was better than nothing.

Unfortunately, sleep, or the lack of it, affects everything about our day: how much energy we have; how cognitively sharp we are; our emotions; our outlook; and our short-term and long-term health, which I wasn't particularly aware of at the time.

And although the on–off sleeplessness I'd lived with for a couple of decades was manageable to a point, after I had three children it became a nightly and unmanageable ordeal. It's not just having children that can snap and scatter your sleep–wake cycle, obviously, but for me this was when things began to fragment seriously. This is hardly surprising given the fractured routines and sleep deprivation that go with the territory of being a parent, but this was not something I had really considered or was in any way prepared for. It just became my norm. First my daughter came along, when I was in my thirties, which made sleep that much harder, and then, less than two years later, what was left of my sleep pattern fell apart when I had twin sons.

Looking back, what really stands out is how debilitating it was. Life seemed overwhelming at times, and my resilience was very up and down. My immune system was clearly shot, too, given the frequent colds, spells of flu and a virus that lingered for months. The lack of energy could be depressing. And the hours spent wide awake in bed were predictable and annoying, to say the least. But then, thankfully, a light went on.

The wisdom of the great-greats

It was early autumn, the nights were closing in and I was reading a book called *So Built We the Wall*, written by my great-great-great uncle, Richard Waters, a pioneer in cognitive therapy and the far-reaching effect thoughts and words can have on our emotions, behaviour and health. I came across his section on insomnia, which inspired me to fix my broken sleep and write this book.

Dick, or Uncle Dick as he was known by friends and family, was a strong, sociable, pipe-smoking character at the heart of the Roaring Twenties. He was also a protégé of the cognitive-therapy poster boy and celebrity guru, Émile Coué – the French pharmacist who coined the catchphrase, 'Every day, and in every respect, I'm getting better and better,' which sparked a global re-think by introducing what was considered back then to be a revolutionary concept centred on self-help and the ability of suggestion to heal. I'd always been vaguely interested in what they both stood for, having grown up with Coué's mantra bouncing around inside my head. But was there anything in those once zeitgeist theories, I wondered? And could they help me to sleep better?

My sleep was worse than ever that autumn, which is why the insomnia segment jumped out at me. Not that I saw myself as 'An Insomniac' with a problem that could be sorted, but rather as someone who would head to bed after a busy day, more than ready for sleep, but then just lie there for hours and hours and hours, unable to drift off. Night after night. And then be shattered during the day.

What had really been getting me down in recent years was that even when I did get enough sleep, from going to bed ridiculously early or playing catch-up with a lie-in, I still woke up feeling exhausted, weak and hollow. If you had offered me another night's sleep, back-to-back, I'd have said, 'Thank you very much' and gone straight back to bed.

There were times when I just hit a wall, burnt out to my core and too weak to do anything except collapse in bed for a day to recharge. Somehow, I hadn't made the connection between all this and the lack of quality sleep I was getting before reading my uncle's book and then delving deeper. The symptoms seemed too extreme, in my defence, although they seem obvious now. And sleep is often underrated. Apart from having my prescription sleeping pills for emergencies, my eye shades, ear plugs and some lavender oil to occasionally sprinkle on my pillow, I just carried on, while sporadically demanding that my doctor run tests for deficiencies and conditions that didn't exist.

Coming across that section on insomnia, however, changed everything – in an instant. My symptoms were not the result of some illness, as I sometimes thought, or the full-on demands of family life, which one doctor had suggested, but the fallout from second-rate sleep that was not doing its job of repairing or energising me to set me up for the day. Officially, I was a chronic insomniac.

Tune out? Or tune in?

When I knew Uncle Dick, he was a warm and gregarious elderly man, with lots of anecdotes to tell, and he still looked after a handful of patients well into his eighties. Having separated from his first wife and lost both his second wife and his son, he was living in a garden flat in Notting Hill, west London, with a bad-tempered African grey parrot that rarely stayed in its cage.

I remember his parrot dive-bombing a childhood friend of mine as she made her way down my uncle's hallway, swooping so low it skimmed her hair and made her shriek, and how it would rush out from its favourite hiding place under a cabinet to peck at my ankles when in a fractious mood.

As a young man, Waters (I'll give him his proper name from now on – it sounds so much more professional than Uncle Dick) was adventurous and fearless, throwing himself into the speed of luge racing while studying at Heidelberg University in Germany. Later, as a professional in London, he wore suits made in Savile Row, hung out at dinner parties and in London pubs, such as the Bunch of Grapes in Knightsbridge, and in the private club-cum-Victorian music hall, the Players' Theatre, which was tucked away in one of the railway arches near Embankment station. He walked with a stick, due to a slight limp that was the result of blood poisoning in childhood, and he spoke with a distinct Dublin–Irish accent, despite living in England for most of his adult life.

We all carry the people we've been close to inside us, no matter whether they are alive or not, which is why, no doubt, I was drawn to Waters' book, in a bid to understand him and what he believed in that little bit more. All his books, and Coué's, had been on my shelves for years, and I have many letters from Coué to my uncle and from Coué's wife, Lucie, who kept in touch after his death, plus Waters' huge leather-bound patient book that details a few of his earlier cases in the opening pages, including letters of thanks.

Waters wrote about sleep and the power of thoughts and words, suggesting that our thoughts affect our body's pre-sleep prep, as does the decision 'I am off to bed'. I thought this was a fascinating idea. But what I wanted to know was: where were we on this 100 years later? Did it hold up with what medics know today? And what had scientists since discovered about the whole world of sleep?

I therefore followed the Coué–Waters thread from then until now and I explored the latest science around sleep, interviewing relevant experts that I discovered along the way. And I tried out everything I learnt on myself: the habit science, light science, neuroscience, experimental psychology, clinical hypnosis, sleep suggestion, everyday sleep solutions ... to see what impact any of it might have on my sleep, energy levels, general health and well-being.

By merging Coué's and Waters' theories with their 21st-century reincarnations and contemporary science, I came to understand sleep issues in a much wider, deeper context. I dismantled my chronic insomnia in the process and set up a strong sleep pattern that I hadn't enjoyed since I was a young child.

Are you sitting comfortably?

Émile Coué discovered the power of words by chance, while working as a pharmacist. He could either hand out medicine to his customers and keep schtum, or he could explain how they worked and sing their praises. The latter would make them that much more effective, he found, thanks to the expectations he implanted in the minds of his clients triggering actual physical change –something that scientists have subsequently shown stands up to scrutiny. And if a customer still wasn't doing too well, he would say, 'What you need is some auto-suggestion. Come for some this afternoon.' The one-to-one suggestion sessions quickly grew into group sessions, and then to packed-out halls around the world. Because what Coué had come to realise was that, unlike contemporary hypnosis, which he dismissed as too vague, he didn't need to put patients to sleep to get physiological results. Simply talking to them about how their condition could improve while they were wide awake worked just as well, by harnessing both the power of suggestion and the placebo effect. He later created his 'every day' mantra (*Tous les jours, à tous points de vue, je vais de mieux en mieux*) so that his method could reach a wider audience.

Coué's feel-good message was a major hit, especially after the horrors of the First World War. Its mix of medicine, suggestion and hypnosis, and its novel self-help Big Idea, were new to society. In contrast to Sigmund Freud, who was working at this time, Coué took total control away from the therapist and put it squarely in the hands of the patient – a self-empowering approach that proved extremely popular with the public, and one he used to treat a wide range of ailments and disorders, including insomnia.

'I am not a healer . . . I am not a magic maker,' wrote Coué, modest as always, when responding to ecstatic praise from his legions of fans, 'My part is to teach [people] what they can do to heal themselves, or at least to improve themselves … using an instrument which we use all our lives long without knowing it – I will say auto-suggestion.' That is to say, to direct the voice inside your head to say things that work to improve your health, and to keep saying them until they cause real behavioural and physical change.

Waters' twist on the Coué method took this one critical step further, arguing that by combining biology with suggestion (and in this case the biology and science of sleep), you can get even greater results through directing the conscious and the unconscious mind. And he was right. The clinical link between mind, brain, body, health and behaviour, including sleep, has since been proven, with this largely untapped area of medicine now being trumpeted as the next frontier, with ground-breaking discoveries in neuroscience to back it up.

Medics, dentists and scientists, who are at the forefront of research today, are using words – just words – to shift physiology, the emotions, body chemicals, mindset and behaviour. They are also using words to boost sleep, health, success, speed recovery, control pain, replace a sense of threat with opportunity and increase performance across the board.

Dr Karen Olness MD, from Cleveland Ohio, for example, had a 50-minute operation on one of her fingers using nothing but hypnosis and self-hypnosis (aka auto-suggestion/self-talk) to kill the pain, with everything filmed to show any incredulous colleagues the power that words alone can have. This was written up in the book that she co-wrote with Daniel P. Kohen, *Hypnosis and Hypnotherapy with Children*. A fake MRI scanner set up by a Canadian university team in 2017 to 'treat' young patients with ADHD achieved long-lasting, measurable results, because the patients were told that it would. While patients at Manchester University NHS Foundation Trust (MFT) are daily talked into a state of restful alertness (deep meditation) to treat extreme physical discomfort as well as sleep issues in a department where patients are given a brief biology lesson to guarantee that the doctors' medical suggestions are effective.

Suggestion, conscious auto-suggestion, self-talk, clinical hypnosis, self-hypnosis, an idea that transforms into action, that voice inside your head – call it what you will. The latest scientific understanding of how this all works, and proof that harnessing it can get dramatic results, both neural *and* physical, means that we can benefit from giving ourselves helpful suggestions in relation to our sleep. By using Waters' spin on the Coué Method alongside sleep science, we can, for example, learn how our sleep-inducing neurons stack up and our brainwaves slow down. We can then improve the quality of our sleep and go to sleep that much more quickly by taking direct action to control our sleep–wake cycle.

Doctor, doctor

Lord Curzon (1859–1925), British politician, art collector and a chronic insomniac, was one of Coué's more high-profile patients and a vocal fan who wrote to the papers to publicise being saved from decades of insomnia by Coué. He also gave payback by introducing Coué to King Albert of Belgium, whom Coué visited several times, cementing the popularity of Couéism in Belgium. Later, when asked about his treatment of Curzon, Coué replied, 'Lord Curzon continues to sleep like a babe.'

Now I would love to know what Coué said to both Curzon and the king, and I just wish that all pharmacists and doctors could have the time and the training to help everyone sleep more easily, especially as it's been estimated that around 30 per cent of the problems that general practitioners face are directly, or indirectly, related to sleep problems. But the sad reality is that sleep is regularly overlooked or not dealt with in any depth.

Although it seems that sleep has always been a problem for some people, not just for the patients of Coué and Waters' era but for different reasons over the centuries, today one of the main issues is that shaving hours off sleep to add on to the day has become typical in what is often a high-octane, high-speed society and a gig economy.

We're kidding ourselves, however, if we think we can barrel through workload pressures, family life or social demands on a drip-feed of caffeine, high-sugar fuel and too little sleep. And why en masse are we not making the connection between this and our sub-standard days and deteriorating health?

Despite the statistics and fear-inducing headlines, sleep issues are said to be under-reported by patients, under-diagnosed or just not recognised as the cause of why people feel as bad as they do and are struggling to fire up or reach their full potential.

The problem is global. Just one in ten Brits talk to their doctor about the dire state of their sleep, despite 30 per cent taking medication to try to deal with it. Every two weeks, more than seven million American drivers nod off at the wheel. And 20 per cent of serious car accidents are put down to sleep deprivation. Up to 70 million Americans suffer from chronic sleep disorders. Around 60 million Chinese suffer from sleep disorders and 45 per cent of Australians say that too little sleep affects their day.

The elderly tend to suffer more than the young, women generally more than men, and low earners more than high earners.

I was one of those one-in-ten Brits who did drag myself round to see my doctor. I would be there one day for a top-up of sleeping pills, which I needed for those times when I was wide awake and increasingly anxious at 3am, or to deal with long-haul jet lag from West Coast America (where my in-laws live) that almost pushed me to the edge. On another day, at a separate appointment, I would be asking my doctor, 'Why do I have no energy?', 'Why do I feel this bad?', 'Why am I always ill', 'Am I anaemic?', 'Do I have a thyroid problem?'. To which various doctors effectively gave a shrug (although various tests were carried out, just to check). But the strange thing is that none of us made the connection between my never-ending symptoms and my inadequate sleep.

The fact is, it doesn't take that much to qualify as an insomniac.

There is short-term acute insomnia, which can last for just days or weeks, and there's chronic insomnia: if you have trouble sleeping three nights or more a week for three months plus, you officially fit the bill. Either way, this will, inevitably, impact your energy, moods, brain power, stress levels, immune system and more.

The problem with calling yourself an insomniac, however (even if your doctor agrees that you are one), rather than just someone who is having trouble sleeping well right now, is that it feels like a done deal: it's part of your identity that you have to live with. Instead, you're better off seeing it as an umbrella term that covers low-grade sleep in general, and as something that might affect you today but doesn't have to tomorrow.

Insomnia is also classified by the American Academy of Sleep Medicine as a subjective disorder. In other words, it's something that comes down to your personal perception of whether or not you have trouble with sleep and if this is having a damaging effect on your day. Perceptions, however, as we'll see later, can be deconstructed and changed – for the better.

Even if you're *not* an insomniac, the majority of us suffer from poor sleep at some point in our lives; some studies find that we all do. And it's not just about the ideal number of hours we're supposed to chalk up. If we want to wake up rested and sidestep the long-term health risks that come with sleep deprivation, we need to get seven to nine *quality* hours. This is all about quality over quantity, as some people bank a decent amount of sleep but still wake up feeling shattered before the day has begun, as I used to. And it's little comfort that those who are officially insomniac often get more sleep than they realise, as they don't feel it, and it certainly isn't quality.

The why behind the how

Having started out with Waters' thoughts on insomnia, the more I read, the more I saw how his method could be applied to so many scientific findings and so many aspects of our lives. I became increasingly aware of just how much control we can have over our bodies, emotions, habits and sleep quality (and more) – using suggestions backed up by science and knowledge, which all comes down to understanding what's going on in our bodies and minds, and working with them – not against them.

Just knowing how habits take shape in the brain, and what we can do to make or break them, allows us to replace an unhelpful sleep pattern for one in which we sleep soundly, for example. Appreciating the effect of daylight and darkness on our health, body chemicals and our sleep makes a very persuasive argument for why we should try to sync in with night and day as much as possible. It's what humans are hard-wired to do. Reframing emotions, a form of suggestion, changes our outlook, our reality and our hormones, which all impact sleep. Reducing stress levels – one of the biggest sleep disrupters – with science-based tactics focused on the mind–body loop, again uses suggestion to boost our happy hormones, defuse stress and allow the sleep-inducing chemistry we need to take place. Even the relationship between diet and sleep is not just about when and what we eat, but also about *how* we eat.

Thanks to Coué and Waters and where they led, I paid more attention to my thoughts and their knock-on effect on my feelings and my sleep, became more aware of stress triggers and the sleep-blocking chemical cascades they set off, and for the first time ever I saw how emotions and reality perceptions could be deliberately changed to benefit my day (and my sleep). I used sleep-supporting suggestions during the day and more biology-based ones at night, to help set off the physiological changes needed for sleep. But I also removed the obstacles lying between myself and sleep and, having made the connection between sleep and our habitual behaviours, I looked at habit science and set up habit cues to create the sleep I was after.

After much research and experimentation, I ended up combining the suggestion and theories of Coué and Waters with 21st-century science, the biology of sleep and the latest in sleep science. This seemed to me to be the only way to understand fully the sleep–wake cycle and, specifically, *my* sleep–wake cycle, and how my habits, mindset, timetable, emotions, body chemicals, stress, and so on, supported or interfered with that. After all, if we don't understand what's stopping us – *personally* – from getting the sleep we need, we can't make the changes needed for us to get a good night's sleep.

Sleep needs to be considered from every angle if we want to upgrade it, taking into account what's happening externally to influence it, but also, crucially, what's going on inside us, in both body and mind.

Your daily creation

One aspect of sleep that is generally overlooked, and which undermines any effort to improve the quality of our sleep, is the biological fact that from the moment we open our eyes in the morning, our sleep countdown is on, because the way we spend our day, hour by hour, directly impacts the quality of our sleep, which in turn controls the quality of our tomorrow.

Cues that help induce sleep build momentum throughout the day, while other cues throw it off course, but both come together to dictate the sleep that we will have later that night: the light/dark signals we surround ourselves with; how long we sleep; whether and when we nap; how much time we spend outdoors, or working, rushing around, stressed out, and at our screens; our daily habits; our body chemicals; and the suggestions we give ourselves.

The quality of our sleep is inseparably woven into our being and our day. It is a product of our biology, behaviour, environment and thoughts – not an add-on that comes out of nowhere as night moves in. And we can support our body's natural, 24-hour sleep–wake rhythms – so that this night–day circle keeps turning effortlessly round and round – by becoming aware of the biology and science of sleep, and understanding, for example, our body's craving for daylight and the darkness of night and what effect this has on us, or how we can change our body chemicals so that we're able to settle into the rest-and-digest state we need to be in to sleep.

Sleep 360

The idea of combining self-talk with the biology and science of sleep might seem strange and unfamiliar, particularly if you're used to experimenting with more standard strategies to help with your sleep, such as decluttering your bedroom, drenching your mornings in sunlight or spraying sleep concoctions into the air at night. This was where I started, too, but what became clear to me early on was that, taken in isolation, the vast majority of sleep methods and top tips out there barely scratch the surface, because there is no quick-fix solution that can rescue our sleep. Even if we throw a handful of strategies and sleep-friendly treats in the direction of our bedroom, they're not going to do that much if we're not looking at the problem from every angle: considering all the causes, not just the symptoms, and recognising that everything about our day feeds into our night.

That's not to say that the decluttering and early morning walks are a waste of energy, as far as your sleep is concerned. Far from it, as I learnt first hand. It's just that all sleep tactics have to be part of a bigger, 360-degree picture, where knowledge and suggestion are key if they're going to have any significant, ongoing effect.

This is where this book comes in. We'll be looking at how those more familiar sleep solutions can be used in a new context for long-lasting results, underpinned by the latest understanding of the science and biology of sleep and how to tailor these tactics to your own personal situation. When it comes to sorting out sleep issues, generic solutions can be far too limited. Understanding the *why* behind sleep science and other relevant areas of science in relation to *your* body and *your* individual sleep–wake pattern is all important.

Do you know why your sleep–wake cycle is in chaos, for example? How to get the body chemicals you need for an excellent night's sleep?

What it takes to break a negative sleep habit? What is keeping you awake at night, or waking you up too early? What is the flip-flop sleep switch and how to activate it? How suggestion can help you sleep? What you can do to get sleep-sabotaging stress chemicals down?

My method looks at sleep in a very different light from usual, but it will help you to understand your sleep patterns in relation to your body, life and mind, and what's going on around you. It focuses on how easily bad sleep habits can become entrenched, and how words can dramatically spike our stress chemicals, which can ruin our sleep. More importantly, it reveals: how biology-based suggestions can reinforce the sleep we need; how we can create desirable sleep habits that last, based on knowing what is going on in our brain; and how our body intuitively tracks the rising and setting of the sun, and why we need to facilitate this. Plus, I've brought together a diverse range of tried-and-tested, science-based tactics that we can use to alter our chemical balance to help carry us off to sleep. All of this gets to the very core of what sleep is about, creating a unique sleep method that is properly effective.

We'll delve into the world of clinical hypnosis, to see how day-to-day self-talk can change our physiology and our sleep. We'll run through the basics of sleep biology so that you're aware of what's going on in your body in relation to sleep, and the far-reaching control you can have over this. We will look at light science and how you can orchestrate the light you need in your day and night; how to create wanted, or dislodge unwanted, sleep habits; how to swap one emotion for another and why this will help you to sleep better; what the most effective stress-busters are that are backed up by science, and how they can drive our stress chemicals down and our well-being and sleep quality up; what are the right foods to eat for the best sleep possible, and when we should eat them; and we'll see why women have a harder time with sleep, depending on where they live in the world, and what they can do about this – and more.

Understanding sleep in this way will allow you to have real control over your sleep, whether you just want to make it deeper and more restorative, or if you have a disruptive sleep issue that's leaving you exhausted and far from your best – or if you're suffering from chronic insomnia, as I was.

And if you're still wondering why just talking to someone, or giving yourself a good talking to, is such a big deal, we'll explore why, from a neuro-scientific perspective, it's the key to cognitive therapy and clinical hypnosis, as well as the way it works to re-write your sleep habits. And we'll discover why, if you can manage to get your brain's attention in this way, changes to your physiology and the same old behaviour can take place.

As I discovered, combining this brain-game technique with sleep science, experimental psychology, habit-building, lining yourself up with the Earth's daily rotation, practical DIY sleep tactics, emotion swaps and some basic biology can be really life-changing. Not only in terms of transforming the quality of sleep – the bedrock of life – but also when it comes to having a better handle on day-to-day life and for overall well-being.

After decades of not being able to sleep easily, going all the way back to my early teens, and far too many nights spent wired and wide awake, and far too many days exhausted, I'm finally able to sleep when I want, and to sleep well, so that when I wake up in the morning I feel rested with plenty of energy to meet the day. There are still some nights when my mind starts whirring as it used to, but not only can I see why this might be happening, I now also have a whole range of tools for dealing with this so that insomnia doesn't step in.

There's a reason Coué's method had him hobnobbing with royalty, and Waters' patients adored him to the end: they were on to something big 100 years ago. And although these two were just my starting point in all this, they made me look at sleep from a very different, 360-degree perspective, where I had to tune in to my mind and body, the bubble I live in, the world around me and the sleep I was getting, to make changes that were going to hit home and last.

Chapter 1

The Illusion of Impossibility

Magic, perception and the power of suggestion – words
that can alter our reality, mind, body *and* sleep.

We might not *like* to think of ourselves as suggestible, but in reality
we are *so* susceptible to suggestion, we'll even believe something that
we're told, despite the fact that it doesn't match up with what's in
front of our eyes – something magicians have been on to for years.
Top magicians run rings round us, curating illusion, perception and
misdirection, exposing how the brain can be tricked into seeing one
thing or another, or not seeing anything at all.

Take a study by Richard Wiseman, magician, author and professor
of the public understanding of psychology, where participants were
convinced that a fake psychic they were watching had succeeded in
making a key bend just because the 'psychic' told them that it was
bending. It didn't bend.

Self-proclaimed 'mentalist and illusionist' Derren Brown, who
declares that he mixes magic with suggestion, psychology, misdirection and showmanship, exploits the power of suggestion by blurring

the lines between the audience's perception of what is going on in front of them and what is actually happening: exposing the secrets behind magic tricks here, but not there; using distraction, suggestion and a well-placed lie; and manipulating attention and awareness to create whichever illusion he's after. He might be controversial as a result of his past efforts to try to persuade people to rob a bank, steal a baby or push a stranger off a high building, and for wrapping magic in the chat of science, but his ability to plant suggestions is there for all to see. Then there's Apollo Robbins, 'gentleman thief' and skilful choreographer of people's attention, who can rob you and remove the cartridge from your pen as soon as look at you, and who is renowned for pickpocketing the American Secret Service, or David Blaine, whose casual levitations leave street audiences gasping.

The reason magicians are able to control and dupe an audience of individual brains is that they play with our assumptions about the things they suggest; we consider their sleights of hand to be impossible – the illusion of impossibility. They also take advantage of our overconfidence in our senses and our ability to see an objective reality.

Why do we accept impossible, pseudo-psychological explanations, such as the idea that a magician can tell which card we chose from a pack by reading our micro-expressions? Because our brains are searching for simple solutions and explanations for what is going on all around us.

But beyond magic tricks and illusions, suggestion, cultural suggestion and self-talk can get results that are not to be sniffed at. And if we are *that* suggestible, whether we like it or not, we might as well use it to our benefit, whether that's to improve our sleep, health or emotional well-being. This was the argument effectively put forward by Coué and Waters all those years ago, and one that is being taken up today by doctors, behavioural scientists, cognitive therapists, experimental psychologists, et al.

So we can switch off that nagging voice inside our mind, which often seems to be working against us, and replace it with another that's more constructive – then keep doing this until it becomes our default setting and the habit sticks, at which point we'll reap the rewards, whether that's greater creativity, professional success, better health or deeper sleep.

You can tell yourself that you're a terrible sleeper – you wake every day at 4am, you're an insomniac – and live with this identity that you have given yourself and fulfil the prophecy. Or you can turn this on its head and tell yourself that your sleep is getting better and better, that you'll sleep more deeply tonight than last night, as if you mean it, preferably out loud (to others, if not yourself). With this suggestion absorbed and transformed into an auto-suggestion, the foundation will be laid for a different thought habit, with different predictions for your brain to follow that will influence your perceptions *and* your behaviour.

Magicians have always been ahead of the game on this subject with their intuitive grasp of how the human brain functions and how easily it can be manipulated to believe different versions of reality. But now scientists and experimental psychologists are increasingly looking at the *why?* behind the *how?*, mining the work of magicians and the illusions they create to gain a greater understanding of how the mind and suggestion work – and how this psychological and physical interchange can be used to advance both science and medicine.

A Canadian team of doctoral researchers exploring this field of medicine at the McGill University is led by former professional magician Jay Olson. In a fascinating research project with wide-reaching medical implications, Olson and his team set up a sham MRI scanner with layers of deception, magician-style, to maximise the power of placebo and the 'external locus of control' (the belief that external influences, such as doctors, are in charge), plus suggestion, perception, expectation and the art of illusion. The programme succeeded in not only making their patients *feel* different, but in achieving real medical results.

Repeated suggestions, as with repeated sleep routines, make their mark, changing habitual thoughts, emotions, physiology and ultimately actions. Coué coined the term 'conscious auto-suggestion' for his wide-awake version of hypnosis and self-hypnosis, which he used to treat any number of complaints, ranging from asthma and acute eczema, to pain, paralysis, digestive issues, depression and insomnia. What Waters did was to take this to the next level, by reinforcing his suggestions with medical insight – a technique, now backed up by 21st-century science, that is gathering momentum.

'Émile Coué was the first to definitely link Mind to Matter; and to demonstrate to the world that disease can be dealt with satisfactorily from a psychological starting point,' wrote Waters. 'The author has done no more than to carry Mon Coué's work to a further stage. That stage is the link between psychology and physiology.'

There's relaxed, and then there's *relaxed*

I'd never been hypnotised before, and even though I knew it would just be a matter of someone talking to me in a lovely, soothing voice – softly popping positive suggestions into my ear – it went far deeper than I expected. Given that this clinical hypnosis session was the modern-day equivalent of what Waters was up to, but being carried out by a doctor, I was intrigued to see what the process involved and what the outcome would be.

I listened and focused and visualised and breathed, as instructed, lying horizontal in a vast reclining leather armchair in a small hospital room where every surface was covered with thank-you cards from patients, with others grouped in frames on the walls. Eyes closed, but awake, I was more than a little self-conscious and ill at ease at first, but I soon became more relaxed than I've ever been. This is called a state of 'restful alertness', where the mind stays awake, but the body melts into the deepest relaxation. By the time I had to surface and open my eyes, some 45 minutes later, I really didn't want to. No massage had ever made me feel quite so calm and weightless. Why would anyone want to snap out of that?

'With hypnotherapy, your perception and thinking process

changes,' explains public health specialist and clinical hypnotherapist
Dr Syed Shariq Hasan at Manchester University NHS Foundation
Trust (MFT), who had talked me into this state of total relaxation.
His patients enjoy a 75–80 per cent success rate for all manner of
disorders, which goes up to 80-plus per cent, with the more receptive under-eighteens. Once you're restfully alert, that's when the
subconscious is most receptive to suggestion and when clinical hypnotherapists can make their medical suggestions to improve your health.

'There are so many functional disorders hypnotherapy can be used
for,' Dr Hasan tells me. It can be used for insomnia, pain, anxiety,
depression, stress, addictions, phobias, unwanted habits (such as nail
biting), panic attacks, chronic fatigue symptoms, teeth grinding,
psychological disorders ... And a functional disorder is anything
we experience that doesn't involve physical abnormalities. As in, it
won't show up in tests. All the sci-fi medical equipment in the world,
for example, can't detect a functional disorder such as a migraine
or insomnia.

We can hypnotise ourselves as well, and we do this with the auto-
suggestions we give ourselves on a minute-by-minute basis (in our
mind or out loud) or using a guided script. It takes 15 to 20 minutes
to induce restful alertness, where we absorb suggestions like a sponge,
and it's a real luxury to have this done by a professional; however,
the things that we tell ourselves throughout the day still mould
who we are. Even a brief insomnia script, such as Waters', or Coué's
proverbial mantra can become instantly relaxing and the repeated
suggestions powerful.

Back in that voluptuous armchair, conscious, but at the same time
so very far removed from the here and now, I visualised oxygen energising every cell in my body when I breathed in, and carbon dioxide being
expelled when I breathed out, with all the stress, tension and past
negatives being rounded up and removed from my body, as suggested
by Dr Hasan. (On pages 182–190 you will find a sleep script written
by him specifically for this book.) And when I reluctantly peeled open
my eyes, forcing myself to engage with my immediate, card-filled

surroundings, I felt stronger and more tranquil, both physically and mentally, than I previously knew possible.

That voice inside your head

It helps if we can get a grip on our reality. What we're focusing on. What we're telling ourselves. And how this can all be shuffled in the blink of an eye. Your reality is not the same as my reality, which is why my memory of something might differ from yours, and why ten witnesses can have ten different takes on a crime scene. All our realities can be putty in our own hands.

One example of how different our side-by-side realities can be, and how suggestions can lodge in our minds and be absorbed by our memories, comes from when I got married in the middle of the French countryside. The plan was that my husband would ride in on a horse, which most guests had been told about beforehand, while I was to turn up in an old Mercedes lent by a friend of a friend. It was all outdoors, under an arch of trees, and there were horses in the next field. But in the end, for a number of reasons, my husband walked in, from a distance, towards the guests. All good, except that, since then, at least three guests have fondly reminisced about how great it was to see him ride in on a horse.

There are many mind-boggling behavioural-science experiments out there that expose how suggestible we all are, whether we're happy about this idea or not, how this suggestibility can transform our reality, and also how it can be exploited to our advantage, changing our body chemicals and how we act.

Even the tiniest self-talk has been shown to get startling results – in a flash – altering how we think, feel, behave and perform, and the physical chain-reactions that go with that; for example, I can tell myself, 'I feel excited', when in fact I feel sick to the stomach with anxiety – and my brain will miraculously buy into this. This comes from a cutting-edge mind–body experiment (more later) that repackages reality to get the best response from the brain. The experiment guaranteed that those taking part achieved top marks when they danced in front of a stranger, gave a persuasive public speech and answered complex maths questions – challenges that usually set off stress and anxiety. Why wouldn't we all want to tap into that? Particularly given that if we can get our stress chemicals down, our sleep will benefit.

The problem is that on a moment-by-moment basis our reality is ruled by our outlook. And most of the things we say to ourselves (in our mind) are negative.

'For most of us, our self-hypnosis is "You really suck at this. You're a really bad person. You don't deserve this." We are usually pretty self-deprecating,' says Dr Laurence Sugarman, director of the Center for Applied Psychophysiology and Self-regulation at the Rochester Institute of Technology, New York State. Dr Sugarman uses bespoke clinical hypnosis in paediatric practice to treat a range of conditions, including autism spectrum disorder, anxiety and asthma, as well as sleep disorders. 'If hypnosis is how we are influenced to drive our psychobiological plasticity,' he tells me, 'being in ruts of the same behaviour over and over again, or on the other hand being really creative and having epiphanies and having new ideas, then our self-hypnosis is not very good.'

Dr Sugarman has also used hypnosis while stitching up the cut of a child who was allergic to anaesthetic, simply by talking to the child and getting her to imagine being on the swings in a playground. Not only did he keep her up to speed with what he was doing as he stitched her up, he suggested that she was healing herself and that she 'turn off the little fountains of blood in her skin, to heal a little better'. In this way, he was able to initiate 'real physiological change'. There's been a great deal of research into the ability of suggestion (aka hypnosis) to decrease bleeding with patients as well as pain and inflammation, among other things, but as Waters, Sugarman and others argue, it's knowing how the body works and what is going on that gets the best results – directing the mind to target these specific areas.

'This is powerful stuff,' Sugarman tells me, speaking from his home in New York State. 'We alter our own endorphin flow. We alter bleeding. We alter blood pressure. We alter thresholds of pain reception. Talk to any triathlete about their use of imagery and focus, driving their metabolism to its absolute limits.'

Olympiads, triathletes and sporty people in general, as we know, use positive go-to mantras, motivational words and other mind–body tactics all the time, to push themselves further and to break through the pain barrier. I even noticed a runner friend of mine doing this to up her game during an informal, though socially competitive, table-football evening, shouting at herself: 'Go on [then her surname]! You can do this!'

The difference is that in this instance we're not running a marathon or heading to the Olympics, or playing table football, we're just trying to improve our sleep. And because sleep is as natural and automatic as breathing, if hurdles aren't thrown in its way, it stands to reason that if elite sportsmen and women can change their reality and performance with a few well-chosen thoughts or words, and if doctors can use this technique to operate on and heal patients, then sleep-friendly self-talk can get results for us, too.

Don't like your reality? How about another?

Reality is a strange fish. Not only is it at the mercy of our hormones (such as whether we feel calm vs stressed), it's also shaped by our habits, suggestion, assumptions and unconscious biases, as well as our focus and priorities, of which we may, or may not, be aware.

In our defence, we're not able to be conscious every second of the day to the workings of our brain. It is processing everything that's happening around us at breakneck speed, drawing our attention to danger or rewards and what we've flagged up as our priorities or of interest. This explains why we can suddenly spin round to find someone staring at us, hear our name in conversation across a crowded room, spot a friendly face in a sea of strangers, or learn a new nugget of information, only to hear frequent references to it in the days that follow. What particularly fascinates researchers, however, is how a specific focus or instruction given to the brain controls our perception of reality and of ourselves, and how this can be so focused that it can be oblivious to something that's jumping up and down right in front of us – even something as big as a gorilla.

With 'the invisible gorilla strikes again' experiment, 24 radiologists were given the familiar task of looking for lung-nodules in a stack of computerised tomography (CT) scans, but what 20 of them failed to spot was a gorilla waving at them from the top corner of a group of scans – a phenomena known as inattentional blindness (IB). To draw even more attention to the impostor, the gorilla image was not only outlined in white, it was the size of a box of matches, more than 48 times the size of a nodule. The radiologists, however, didn't see it, because they hadn't given their brains the task of looking for a gorilla. Their concentration and focus were elsewhere. This follows on from, and was a deliberate homage to, the notorious 'invisible gorilla' video experiment that came out of Harvard University. Six people were filmed passing round a basketball while viewers were given the job of counting the number of passes made by those wearing white (www.theinvisiblegorilla.com – spoiler alert: you might want to watch the link, before reading further). What 50 per cent of those taking the test failed to notice was a person dressed as a gorilla who walked through the middle of the group, paused, turned and beat their chest directly to camera, before moving on. Impossible to miss, you would have thought, looking at the footage, but magic tricks, as we know, work in the same way: we're so busy focusing on our chosen priority (or wherever the magician is directing our focus) that we're completely blind to the sleight of hand that's taking place right under our noses.

Our brain is also playing catch-up – constantly. And that further messes with our reality. Why? Because there's a one-tenth of a second time lag between what we see and that information making its way to our brain and, in order to deal with it, our brain makes an educated guess to predict the future. It's not a tactic that's always helpful, or accurate.

Dr Gustav Kuhn's 'vanishing ball trick' is one of the many experiments he devised to demonstrate how misdirection can make us see things that are not in front of us, or fail to see others that are. In the trick a magician throws a ball into the air three times, but the third time it doesn't fall back down. Baffling, except that it turns out that the magician didn't actually throw the ball up in the air the third time, he simply moved his hand as if he was throwing it, and the brain, knowing what had come before and guessing what would come next, filled in the rest.

Splashed across gentleman thief Apollo Robbins's website is: 'It's not what you look at that matters. It's what you see.' As with everyday life, our version of reality and how we read situations is likewise based on what we see – be that the negatives or the positives directed our way, the blue sky or the grime, problems or solutions, the scowl you think you saw or the compliment given, the triggers for disrupted sleep or insomnia, or the cues, suggestions and changes that can overturn it. As shown with the gorilla experiments, we can consciously choose what to focus on in our daily lives to manipulate our reality, what we prioritise, how we feel about different situations and how we see ourselves.

Focus your brain and you orchestrate your day

'We create our own experience,' says executive mind coach and cognitive hypnotherapist, Kirsty Macdonald, when we meet to talk. 'There is *nothing* that we experience as human beings that we are not setting up for ourselves. We're doing it all and we just believe the stories. So you need to upgrade the story and tell yourself one that supports who you want to be, rather than one that undermines it. Build it and they will come: "I am someone who can sleep easily. I might not be sleeping easily right now, but I *am* someone who sleeps easily." You can tell yourself that this is factually true. It's not a lie: "I might not have slept that well to this point, but I am a human being who can sleep easily." It is possible to change things. The brain is not fixed.'

What are the messages and focus you're giving yourself on a daily basis that shape your reality? Are they unhelpful, undermining, self-fabricated? If so, bin them. Because if the conscious mind and the unconscious mind are taking their lead from these pointers and honing in on them to create your perception of reality, and you're telling yourself and everyone else that you only ever sleep for five or six hours, you're a chronic insomniac, you wake at 2am every night, you lie awake for hours, you wake exhausted, you barely sleep a wink, this is what your unconscious will take as read and helpfully serve up on a platter. Also, as Peter Whorwell, professor of medicine and gastroen-terology at the Manchester University NHS Foundation Trust (MFT) points out to me, your *perception* of how well you do or don't sleep also affects how you feel the next morning – rested, or not – regardless of how much sleep you may have actually had.

Instead, you can change the incoming message. As with positive sleep comebacks recommended by cognitive therapists and practised by cognitive hypnotherapists, you can consciously feed yourself lines such as, 'I've slept badly for years, but tonight I'm going to sleep much better than last night,' and let your unconscious chew on that. If the movie in your mind is destroying you, swap the reel.

I did this very deliberately when I realised how easily reality can be reconfigured. Instead of lamenting the fact that I couldn't get to sleep for hours, or had slept dreadfully the night before, I started telling myself and (sometimes) those around me that: I was going to get to sleep much faster than before and that the quality of my sleep was improving because of all the changes I was making; by tuning into my body, I was now working with it to sort out my sleep, manipulating my physiology, body chemicals and emotions, and that this was removing one of the biggest obstacles to sleep, hyper-arousal; by anchoring my mornings in daylight, I was helping my sleep drive and circadian clocks to do their thing; and that the scientifically based changes I'd made to my sleep habits, routine and bedroom had ruptured my old habits and buried them deep . . .

It's a trick of sorts. A trick that allows you to halt your unconscious auto-pilot in its path, tell it a different story and set it running off in a different direction, and it's a trick that neuroscientists are exploring ever more deeply with some useful and mind-bending results. Take the research into how the physiological symptoms that come with stress are so similar to those that come with excitement that the two can be flipped. As Coué put it, '[the unconscious mind] is credulous and accepts with unreasoning docility what it is told', but especially so, it turns out, when what you're saying makes physiological sense.

What's willpower got to do with it?

In all of this, our imagination can be our worst enemy, setting off anxiety and a physiological cascade in response to imagined fears/horrors/failings/hours of sleeplessness that possibly do – or possibly don't – lie somewhere in the future, and which can become our reality, as a very real, self-fulfilling prophecy. But what we need to remind ourselves is that future fear (or not-so-future fear) is just the imagination running wild before anything has actually happened. Instead, by disarming anxiety, or channelling it somewhere useful and directing the voice and images inside your mind, you can cut your stress levels and tame an out-of-control imagination that is setting you up as a hopeless sleeper, destined to be sleep-starved for the rest of your life – and in the process change your reality.

Imagine walking along a plank of wood at ground level. No problem. Now, will yourself to walk along one suspended between the summits of two cathedral towers. 'What's in control?' Coué loved to ask his patients. Is it your conscious will, urging you forward with rational argument, or your imagination that sees you plummeting to a grizzly end? The imagination is clearly in control. Our inbuilt fight-or-flight mechanism is sparking into action to guard us against the imagined danger. That's. Its. Job.

But what if the fears are irrational, habitual or ingrained, such as the fear of not being able to get to sleep? Or the imagined bedroom associations that conjure up hours of wired, bug-eyed, stressful, stomach-churning insomnia? The fear of not being able to do something we're perfectly capable of? The fear of messing up a new job (impostor syndrome)? The fear of not being able to drive on a high-speed road? The list is endless. And the more we think about it, the more we accept and anticipate this fear, making it a reality before it's even happened.

I used to have this with sleep – the image of myself lying wide awake for hours, unable to fall asleep, which was my reality – until I dismantled my sleep habits and my sleep images and built up some new ones in which I sleep like a log. You might have noticed your imagination doing similar things. Have you ever found yourself in the middle of doing a task, action or challenge, even quite a minor one, without question, until you suddenly doubt yourself and wobble? Is that over-protective imagination or habitual, undermining auto-suggestion?

Either way, we're 'wretched puppets of which our imagination holds all the strings. We only cease to be puppets when we have learned to guide our imagination,' as Coué wrote, adding:

> Contrary to what is taught, it is not our will that makes us act, but our imagination. If we often do act as we will, it is because at the same time we think that we can. The more a person with insomnia determines to sleep, the more excited he becomes; the more we try to remember a name which we think we have forgotten, the more it escapes us (it comes back only if, in your mind, you replace the idea: 'I have forgotten', by the idea 'it will come back'); the more we strive to prevent ourselves from laughing, the more our laughter bursts out. We must then apply ourselves to directing our imagination which now directs us; in this way we easily arrive at becoming masters of ourselves.

Although we might not be able to force sleep, we can very deliberately and effectively cultivate it by knowing its biological building blocks and clearing any obstacles that are in the way: confused sleep habits and associations, rotten auto-suggestions, a persistent identity attachment to being insomniac, out-of-sync circadian clocks, an environment that's sabotaging our efforts to sleep, a hyper-aroused mind, chaotic chemicals, and so on. And with all of that under control and the right cues (and rewards) in place, we can ditch counting sheep and adopt a new, suggestive mantra that speaks to our imagination with the power to alter our physiology and our reality: 'I am going to sleep now ...'

Biologists, one and all

Waters, who brought the Coué method to the attention of London's fashionable crowd in the 1920s, first diagnosed what was wrong with his patients and then gave them a simple biology lesson: a rundown on how their healthy body should be working (rather than how it was not working) before offering up suggestions for the mind and autonomous nervous system to act upon. To do this, he would sit on the arm of their chair, talk quietly into their ear, and even tell them that they didn't have to listen if they didn't feel like it, as their subconscious was taking it all in.

He didn't believe in raking over the past, or dredging the psychological side of things, as Freud and others were doing at this time. Instead, he pinpointed what was not functioning as it should and went from there. As for insomnia, Waters wrote an auto-suggestive script for patients to read to themselves or have read to them to train themselves to sleep well through methodical repetition (see Chapter 9).

Professor Peter Whorwell uses a technique very similar to that of Waters, combining suggestion with an understanding of biology (tell the brain what the body needs to do, and then let it do its thing), so that his patients can change what's going on in their bodies for the better, with dramatic medical results that have been endorsed by the National Institute for Health and Care Excellence (NICE).

Whorwell gives his patients a very basic and straightforward tutorial in the body mechanics surrounding their disorder and how these can be made to run smoothly, before using 'gut-focused hypnosis' to treat a range of incapacitating bowel disorders, including the most common gastrointestinal disorder, irritable bowel syndrome (IBS), a debilitating illness affecting 8 million people in the UK and an estimated 25–45 million in the United States.

Although sufferers are often dismissed as having 'only IBS', Whorwell points out that nearly 40 per cent of the patients referred to him are suicidal because no one else has been able to help them, and their suffering is so intense that they are struggling to hold down jobs and relationships, let alone have any quality of life. On top of this, *all* his patients complain that they sleep badly and are constantly exhausted, although tests have shown that this is more to do with their perception of how well they sleep rather than how they actually sleep.

Hypnosis, Whorwell tells me when I visit him in his hospital department, is nothing more than talking to someone in a different way. There's nothing sinister going on, no loss of control or consciousness. It's just a means of communication that can calm people down and make them feel relaxed. By introducing positive suggestions using Whorwell's technique, patients direct their attention to specific areas of their body, helping them to visualise all the cogs in the wheel and how they can make their body function as it should.

'It's a shame that a technique which is incredibly powerful is allowed to be used for entertainment purposes,' says Whorwell. 'I get patients who say, "Am I going to behave like a chicken?", baggage that's a real problem to get rid of. Hypnosis is not like it's portrayed in the movies or in the media, or on the television. This is a powerful technique which is teaching you to control your body, rather than your body controlling you. You will be more in control of your body and, if you want, other things. You will be able to control your stress levels. You will be able to control how your life goes, because your body and mind are more in tune, and your whole body will benefit from this.'

Your brain has got this

Professor Whorwell wasn't always convinced by hypnosis. He was on the lookout for anything that might help patients who had otherwise reached the end of the line and he thought it was worth a punt. *It might at least relax the gut*, he reasoned.

But it did more than that. Although straight hypnosis didn't achieve a great deal, Whorwell tells me, the biology-based clinical hypnosis he went on to develop, where the mind is trained to focus on what the body needs to do to improve its health (along the lines of Waters), was an incredible success. It had a 75–80-plus per cent response rate, meaning that 75–80-plus per cent of his patients were now in control of their symptoms when all other medical treatments had failed them.

Lab tests have backed this up: his team's use of medically grounded hypnosis gets biological results that can actually be measured. Even more importantly, they are results that last, such as reducing pain by turning down hypersensitivity in the body. As Whorwell explains, 'If you hypnotise people and tell them not to feel pain, the anterior cingulate cortex, where the emotional content of pain is processed, is down-regulated. It doesn't glow as much. That suggests that hypnosis is changing the way you process pain. The pain comes to your brain, but your brain can deal with it. We're helping patients at the cerebral level but also at the local level: making the gut less sensitive, but when the pain still gets up there, the brain's not as sensitive. It's not so reactive. The thinking behind it is that we have a functional disorder. There's no structural abnormality there, so the thing is a disorder rather than a disease. Nothing irreversible going on. So can we teach the patient to reverse it and make it work? The power of the mind over the gut and that sort of thing.'

The power of the placebo

There are, of course, parallels to be drawn with the placebo effect – when sugar pills have been found to improve memory and cognitive performance, and bring down blood pressure, reduce pain and effect real physiological change – and a placebo 'scent' (explained in 'Memories inhaled' on pages 111–112), which has been used to trigger creativity. Both are effective thanks to the individual's *expectation* that the medicine, or scent, would have this effect. In fact, *all* medicines rely on the placebo effect to get the results that they do. And even honest placebos get significant results, despite the fact that the patient knows full well that what they're taking is a placebo.

One major difference between placebo and the technique practised by Whorwell's department, he points out, is that his clinical technique not only hits home, it stays put: 'Presumably what we're doing is harnessing the placebo effect and making it last, rather than this transitory phenomenon that you lose after three, four months. And with the studies we've done – long-term studies – we know it lasts.' Very occasionally, somebody might fall by the wayside, he says, in which case Whorwell's team just gives them a top-up clinical hypnosis session or two.

Professor Whorwell, as with Waters (who always insisted his patients be under the care of a medically trained doctor), sees clinical hypnosis as just one part of a therapeutic package to be used alongside conventional medicine and diagnostics, and not as a standalone treatment. And he, too, has found that raking over possible psychological skeletons in the cupboard is not necessary to get results. Clinical hypnotherapy is not used to focus on the past, leaving patients with exhumed and rekindled memories and emotions to deal with, as some therapies do. Instead, patients are given an elementary biology talk-through, specific to their disorder, followed up with 12 weekly sessions of wide-awake hypnosis. During those sessions they are induced into that state of restful alertness, using a number of techniques, including progressive muscular relaxation, where they are introduced to the power of the mind growing stronger and stronger and stronger, to the point where the mind can control the body, rather than the body controlling the mind – a process that is repeated to the patient over and over again.

Patients are sent away with an audio recording of a post-hypnotic script, made by their therapist, to listen to on a daily basis to keep them on track and to firmly lodge the suggestions that have been made to them. And although these are designed to focus on their gut symptoms, to relieve their suffering, the scripts also help them to sleep better by making them more relaxed.

Self-hypnosis is also very effective, without a one-to-one with a therapist, says Whorwell, as long as the voice is right for the patient – a sound that they find melodious and hypnotic. Calm and soothing – audio velvet.

The other half of the equation

Core exhaustion, blinding headaches, inexplicable pain and tingles – there's no denying we can be test-crazy these days in the West. When debilitating symptoms take hold, we head to the doctor for blood tests and the rest. Is there a brain tumour? A thyroid problem? Cancer? But state-of-the-art medical equipment and tests draw a blank, unless there's a structural disease, something that's biologically visible under the microscope. And where does that leave us? Being told 'You're fine. The scan's clear. Move along' doesn't mean the symptoms and the discomfort are not there, or that the extreme tiredness will go away.

I insisted on having quite a few blood tests over the insomniac years, convinced that I must have a deficiency of some sort that would explain my total exhaustion. Nothing showed up. But, as I have discussed, functional disorders don't flash up with a treatable cause, no matter how many tests and diagnostics you put yourself up for.

Western medicine's diagnose-and-treat approach can, of course, get extraordinary results. But it's also the reason the US has been rocked by an epidemic of opioid overdoses, because the majority of opioid abusers started their trajectory with prescriptions. The argument increasingly being put forward in the medical world is that if an individual has the ability to help themselves, on some level, to make mainstream medicine that much more effective, or to help patients become less drug dependent, surely we're letting ourselves down by ignoring the potential that is inside all of us?

As Dr Sugarman tells me, 'From a Western, medical, allopathic point of view, we think that medication is wonderful and powerful, and isn't it great what we can do with medications? What if it's always been true that we are the other half of that equation? Why aren't we encouraging every child with asthma to learn about the power of breathing, heart rate variability, autonomic regulation, and how their body works, because these can be really powerful ways to counter the effects of asthma?'

Opting for a more dual-action approach, combining conventional medicine with something that's been around for hundreds of years (for example, the power of suggestion, clinical hypnosis, the health benefits of placebo, experimental psychology), as many doctors and scientists are now doing, taps into the mind's ability to make life-changing psychobiological changes, including tackling insomnia. Because not only can we change to our advantage what our inner (and outer) voice is saying – or at least give it a slap on the wrist whenever it gets too negative or undermining – we can re-write our reality by taking control of our imagination, and we can also use what we know about the biology of sleep to help us get the quality sleep we need.

Nothing to do with zombies

There's no denying that hypnosis and self-hypnosis have had a bad press over the years. Not only has hypnosis been culturally misrepresented with swinging watches and zombie trances, often mixed up with Franz Mesmer's 'animal magnetism' and mesmerism, but also there has been a lack of clear understanding of what it is and what it isn't, and a lack of consensus on the right terms to use. That Hypnos was the god of sleep in Greek mythology probably hasn't helped.

Scottish surgeon James Braid (1795–1860), who is recognised as the father of hypnosis and hypnotherapy, apparently regretted choosing the misleading word 'hypnosis' because of its link to sleep. He described hypnosis as nothing more than 'concentrated attention and various forms of suggestion' – nothing to do with humiliating stage hypnosis or a loss of self-control. Ninety per cent of his patients said that they felt awake throughout, only 10 per cent were going somewhere deeper. 'I have already stated the wonderful power of the human mind, when inward consciousness is strongly directed to any part of a sensitive person, in changing physical action,' wrote Braid.

As for sleep, suggestion wrapped up in a script and the constant self-hypnosis of self-talk is made infinitely stronger by a knowledge of sleep science and what needs to be going on in your body for you to sleep well. It is a critical part of a surround-sound body-balancing package that can be used to alter our perceptions, neural pathways, habits, outlook, expectations, body chemicals and the quality of our sleep.

As Sugarman's work and Whorwell's department have conclusively demonstrated, Waters' take on the Coué method that combines suggestion with biology gets long-term medical results where straight hypnosis doesn't. By understanding the science and biology of sleep, we can use sleep-based suggestions to initiate the physiological changes we need to sleep well today and in the future.

From biology to bed

I started listening to Waters' short sleep script, which I had recorded on my phone, very early on in this process. It helped me to change my attitude towards sleep and to prepare mentally each evening: to unwind before bed and to draw a line between the pace of thought needed during the day compared to that at night.

The constant, repetitive message embedded in the script sent a clear, unequivocal signal to my brain about the expected sleep count-down ahead, and how my mind and body would relax and change for 'ever more complete, full and restful sleep', helping to alter my sleep, thought and behaviour habits thanks to the repeated suggestions I heard every day.

With time and knowledge, I often added a mini self-hypnosis session at night, to help stop my whirring mind, and I still do this when needed. All this involves is some slow, deep breathing to get into a more meditative state, and then a gentle reminder of what is, or should be, going on in my body – a state of rest and digest, slow brainwaves, sleep-inducing chemicals – the physiological changes needed for sleep, helped along with a few deliberate, biology-based suggestions.

I might also remind myself of the blurred line between being awake and asleep (see Chapter 2), which takes away the pressure to chase sleep, as well as about the flip-flop sleep switch (see page 43), which is inevitably activated to turn off our conscious state as we get sleepier, the biology of which I will describe in the next chapter.

When wide awake and active, dealing with my day, I took note of everything that was impacting my sleep–wake pattern – daylight and the night sky, and their control over my melatonin levels, or how a pause, however brief, was helping to bring down daily stress and its sleep-disrupting chemicals – in order to keep my sleep on course. I also took on Dr Sugarman's description of self-hypnosis – that constant self-talk that might be saying, 'You really suck at this. You're a really bad person' – and challenged any thoughts that were activating the sleep-sabotaging stress chemicals, as well as any that were dictating future insomnia.

The increased self-awareness that has come with researching all this has been incredibly enlightening and empowering, and it makes me wonder how I managed before without this insight. If we can appreciate just *how* suggestible the human brain is, we can consciously and deliberately choose to use words that spark real physical, chemical change and work magic to transform how we feel, behave and sleep for the better. Or we can choose not to.

---

4 top tips

1. Accept how suggestible the brain is and make this work for you.
2. Switch sleep-sabotaging thoughts for ones that set you up as a solid sleeper.
3. Use biology-based sleep suggestion to change your perceptions, physiology and sleep patterns.
4. Listen to a suggestive sleep script (as I will explain in Chapter 9), to help rewrite your sleep thought habits.

Chapter 2

Life Beneath Your Skin

How is it that we can slow our brainwaves down
and nudge ourselves to sleep?

The Maharaja of Alwar, famous for his fabulous wealth and love of
Rolls-Royces, was so taken by the Coué Method, which was all the
rage in the 1920s, that he invited Coué back to India with him after a
trip to Europe, offering to set up a tour for him at the other end. 'But
though the idea was abandoned so far as Coué himself was concerned,
the Maharajah [sic] took other steps to assist in the spread of Couéism,'
wrote Orton in his book *Émile Coué: The Man and His Work* (1935).
He doesn't mention that Coué, in turn, asked Richard Waters to go
to India on his behalf in a letter he wrote to him in 1923.

As it turned out, Waters did not travel to India as the Maharaja's
guest, for reasons that have been lost to time, but which no doubt
would have pleased Orton, whose book attempts to set himself up
as Coué's natural successor, but the relationship between Coué and
Waters had clearly been cemented. Whereas Coué's fame led him to
simplify treatment to his catch-all proverbial phrase, backed up by his

bestseller and lectures in packed-out halls that enabled him to reach bigger and bigger audiences, Waters' more local success saw him stick with tailor-made one-to-one sessions where he focused on clinical suggestions specific to the individual's needs.

He wasn't interested in his patients' past, as previously mentioned, because he worked from the point where people were in the present, physically and mentally, but he found that they usually wanted to tell him their life story, so he sat puffing on his pipe for the first consultation, which cost five guineas, listening without interruption, saying at the end, 'From now on we will not talk about the past.'

Waters had an uncanny knack for diagnostics, according to his professors at medical school, having started out studying medicine in Dublin before being drawn to Coué's practice in the north-east of France. After questioning his patients, he arrived at an understanding of the problem and what needed to be put right, although if it was a matter that needed medical treatment, he sent them straight to a doctor, so that the two treatments could work side by side.

By combining biology with suggestion, much like Professor Whorwell, Dr Sugarman, Dr Hasan and others, Waters helped his patients to help themselves, earning himself a loyal following and successfully treating a whole range of conditions ranging from tuberculosis to serious skin complaints, pre-exam anxiety, depression and insomnia – the idea being that if your brain can focus on the biology of sleep, for example, you can give everything an insider's nudge in the right direction.

When it came to sleep, Waters also recognised what scientists have since proven: that sleep has nothing to do with rest when it comes to the brain and autonomic (auto-pilot) nervous system that keeps your heart beating and your lungs breathing. Instead, it is busy repairing damage and preparing us for the day ahead.

'Sleep is not rest if rest is understood as inertia or idleness,' he wrote. 'A sleeping body has work to do just as a waking one has. It is different work in the main, but it is all important and must be well and truly carried out if we are to awaken fresh and ready for the day.'

Sleeping on the job

Scientists might not know everything (yet) that goes on in the brain when we're asleep, but they do know that Waters was right when he said that there's no inertia in sleep. The brain is extremely active: about 75–80 per cent active, it's believed, busy processing memories and flushing out potentially hazardous neurotoxic waste that's built up during the day.

With an estimated 86–100 billion neurons (nerve cells) and an equal number or more of glial 'housekeeping' cells crammed into the human brain, which give us the most complex of communication networks buzzing with electrochemical signals, it goes without saying that the brain doesn't have an off button. It does, however, have the ability to dull our aroused awake state and to douse us with the sleepy hormone melatonin and other shut-down triggers. Which means that one minute we're conscious and the next we're not.

Brain exploration is still in full swing, but scientists know more than enough to track what's going on in there as we prepare for sleep and finally nod off. It's having a grasp of this biological world beneath the surface, even if it's just a hazy, lay-person understanding of what's going on – and what *should* be going on – in the brain and body's wake–sleep cycle that can help you to get the results you're after.

Absorb the biology and the neuroscience, argued Waters, and you feed your body and mind the priorities you want it to work on. 'We explain to the patient the cause and nature of his trouble,' wrote Waters, describing how he treated patients. 'We produce in his mind a full understanding of the purpose of our suggestion. Then we complete our sitting, by giving him a suggestion that sums up for him what we have taught, as well as explaining and impressing our meaning on his imaginative consciousness.' Suggestions were also sometimes given in the form of a script that worked to bolster and lodge the message.

Likewise, the sleep biology round-up in this chapter will give you the window you need so that you can direct your mind, body and sleep using biology-based suggestions. As Professor Whorwell puts it, 'Teach patients to help themselves.'

A stand-off that's easily won

From the moment we wake up, a starting gun is fired. Although rested (ideally) when we first crawl or leap out of bed – whether we are a night owl or morning lark (depending on our chronotype) – as the day progresses, an internal sleep drive gathers strength. During this time, a build-up of the chemical adenosine, if left undisturbed, makes us increasingly tired and ready for bed.

Hand in hand with this, signals from all around generate a night-and-day rhythm that carries us in the same direction. The signals of light, temperature, time, social and work calendars combined with our body chemicals, central nervous system, gut and circadian body clocks should *all* be synced and working together. (Our circadian rhythm is a roughly 24-hour pattern that exists in all our cells, with fluctuating blood pressure, body temperature and sleep–wake cycle depending on the time of day.) In this way our body clocks make sure that when it's time to sleep, both the body and mind are ready to let nature do its thing. Although, of course, if our body clocks are out of whack, our sleep will be upended, which we'll explore in depth in the next chapter.

If everything is synced, this is when something known as the flip-flop switch comes into its own. With the body's sleep drive having gathered momentum throughout the day, and the brain now powering down as we unwind, once the lights are out, our sleep-prompting chemicals should be at maximum strength with everything starting to fragment slightly. This is the tipping point when the battle between the neurons trying to keep us awake and those trying to get us to sleep is won by the sleepy side, and we go to sleep – in a matter of minutes.

The flip-flop switch

This rapid shift from being awake one moment to asleep the next is called the flip-flop switch, as with the switches found on an electrical circuit that guarantee a fast and total transition from one state to another. The way it works in the brain is that there's effectively a face-off between the sleep-inducing cells and those programmed to keep us awake, until the neurons on one side overwhelm their opponents on the other, and the switch is flicked.

Without this switch, we'd be constantly moving back and forth, in and out of sleep, throughout the day and night, and would spend most of our time in a bit of a daze. All of this explains why those suffering from chronic sleep deprivation can go to sleep at any time there's an opportunity for a sleep top-up, as their sleepy neurons are already stacked high, and why narcoleptics can fall asleep in the middle of any wide-awake activity, as a result of damage to this switch, which stops it from staying in place.

The eyes have it

When it comes to the pre-flip-flop crunch, this is where last-minute direct action can help you get to sleep faster. The hypothalamus, a small but powerful part of the brain, effectively flicks another switch to deactivate certain cell groups in the thalamus and the cerebral cortex that keep us alert. And this part of the sleep cycle comes down to light, or the lack of it.

Before deciding whether or not to launch a sleep-inducing chemical cascade, the circadian clocks in the hypothalamus and pituitary take stock of the surrounding light using receptors in the eyes to see what action it should take. If it's bright, light and full of blue-white screens, forget sleep. You're staying awake. The arousal circuit is reading the stay-awake signals and will fire up accordingly, whether or not it's over-riding the sleep drive within.

By contrast, if it's dark out there, the hypothalamus will action the chemicals needed to sleep. By dispatching melatonin and the amino acid GABA, it shuts down the state of arousal that comes with being awake, allowing your brainwaves to start shifting down a gear or two. GABA, a chemical messenger that's only activated in the evening and is an inhibitory neurotransmitter, carries this shut-down message from neuron to neuron, helping us to relax and dampening our wide-awake, excitable arousal circuitry.

By blacking out your bedroom, eliminating light pollution and opening your eyes when you lie in bed, so that your retinas and brain can absorb the darkness, you can power this sleep-chemical reaction and beef up your sleep-inducing neurons with each passing minute (more on this in Chapter 3).

An old-fashioned cocktail

Cortisol, dopamine, oxytocin: to say that I was more or less oblivious to my body chemicals in the past, and the control they have over me, is a massive understatement. I really couldn't have told you the difference between any of them, let alone how to control them, give them a boost – or the opposite – to shift the mix in my favour. But the fact of the matter is that the chemical cocktail inside us not only defines our daily personality but also the quality of our life, health *and* how we sleep.

This was another of Waters' big passions. Our endocrine system – our glands and their hormones – are who we are, affecting our personality 'to an extraordinary extent', he lectured. Which is one reason why too little sleep can leave us cloaked in a sleep-hungry personality – scratchy, quick to overreact, and not the sharpest. 'I got out of bed on the wrong side' is one way of putting it.

There's also a breakdown in communication that takes place between the part of the brain that's in charge of our emotional responses (the medial pre-frontal cortex) and our emotional HQ (the amygdala) when we're low on sleep, which adds fuel to the fire of this sleep-short identity. And when these two areas of the brain are not talking to each other (such as when they're out of sync), as they are with a lack of sleep, we're left on a short emotional fuse where we can lose control of our emotions and react to minor problems and irritations as dramatically as we would to major ones. All of which has been linked to not getting enough REM (rapid-eye movement) dream sleep (more on that on pages 50–51), something that I was at the mercy of for far too long.

It's no surprise, when you think about it, that those of us who struggle with sleep tend to have excessive levels of cortisol hurtling around our bodies during the day *and* when we head to bed at night. That's cortisol, the action hormone, the one we need to get us out of bed in the morning and which is also related to stress, *not* 'the hormone of darkness', sleep-inducing melatonin. It's little wonder that the body can't settle into a seamless shut-down with all those get-up-and-go chemicals being pumped around your system. Even if you put sleep to one side for a moment, no one wants that much cortisol hanging around day or night, as it's been linked to major chronic diseases, lower immune function, higher blood pressure and cholesterol, weight gain, depression and more.

As a result, I now try to keep my chemicals more balanced during the day so that I can be more the person I want to be (in other words, less cortisol makes you less stressed and vice versa). I know that if I head to bed overloaded with cortisol, I'll have a bad time waiting for it to subside before my sleep drive can take off and my sleep-inducing neurons pile up high enough to tip the scales.

The three top sleep wreckers in the Sleep Council's Great British Bedtime Reports are: stress (approx. 50 per cent), partners (25 per cent) and noise (20 per cent). With this in mind, I have a whole range of practical stress-busting techniques backed up by science to help keep my stress chemicals in check (see 'Stress-busters' on pages 122–123). Having an understanding of sleep biology and how effectively this can be combined with self-talk, as well as a knowledge of some sleep science and my body chemicals (how they are triggered and what I need them for in different situations), has been a real eye-opener that has transformed my sleep into something that I have control over rather than something I just have to live with, no matter how bad it gets.

Your personal stress-response team

As mission control for some of our most vital hormones, the main job of the hypothalamus in the brain is to keep the body's status quo on track, by regulating our sleep patterns, stress levels, body temperature, weight, emotional responses, blood pressure, growth, moods, thirst and sex drive – otherwise known as homeostasis. It has a whole bunch of jobs to do, wrapped up in our behaviour and unconscious (autonomic) body mechanics.

Also, by joining forces with the pituitary 'master' gland and the adrenal gland, the hypothalamus is part of a powerful trio – the HPA axis – which makes up our automatic brain–body stress-response team. This creates a potent neuroendocrine triangle and a feedback loop that links our nervous system, brain, spinal cord and endocrine system.

By keeping a sharp eye on our electro-chemical reactions to feelings and environmental triggers and anything that is affecting us, our HPA stress-response team work together to produce the chemicals it estimates we need to deal with the situation we're in (which is how our body chemicals can end up ruling us).

Whether you're feeling stressed, wound up, worried, on edge, anxious, primed to fight or flight, your HPA axis has your back and is ready to respond to the threat, whether real or imagined: your pituitary, thyroid and adrenal glands are all set to flood the system with 'action' chemicals, such as cortisol and noradrenaline (also known as norepinephrine). This is great if you need an instant shot of adrenaline (epinephrine) to deal with whatever challenges are being hurled your way, but it's the last thing you need if you're trying to go to sleep. And if your stress levels are out of control (with or without you being fully aware of them), the action chemicals will just keep coming.

Stress is that moment when our body's automatic, primal fight-or-flight response kicks in, ready to save us from the perceived danger that's threatening us by stressing us out: it makes the heart beat faster, increasing blood pressure, blood sugars, and the fats necessary for extra energy and helpful action hormones, leaving us alert and both mentally and physically primed for any rapid-response survival action that's needed. With day-to-day stress, however, we're not in any real physical danger – such as being chased by a wild animal or a hostile person – we're just under attack in a different way. But it's enough to block fight or flight's opposite, rest and digest, the state we need to be in to sleep easily.

Waking up throughout the night is a problem of sleep fragmentation, or sleep maintenance, and is called 'wake after sleep onset' (WASO), which is often brought on by stress. Not being able to fall asleep easily is known as delayed sleep-onset latency (SOL). And then there's early morning awakening, which can also be triggered by stress, worries, depression or an overload of work, for example. The problem is that even once any stress or negative trigger has gone from our life, habitual sleep patterns such as these can carry on regardless if we don't take action to set them right. But if we can allow our stress-response team to step down for the night, we open the door for the sleep-activating chemicals our bodies need.

Who are you calling hyper-aroused?

All in all, the more scientists learn about the body and mind, the more Coué and Waters' theories bear out that both body and mind are one, and that neither can be treated as a stand-alone. With body clocks, self-talk and stress under control, and with GABA and melatonin levels where they need to be, we can actively help our sleep-inducing neurons to win the battle and flick the flip-flop switch. Breathing slows down, brainwaves become less compressed, body temperature drops, the calming parasympathetic nervous system steps up, and this relaxed state carries us off to sleep – unless you classify, officially, as an insomniac.

Those who are medically recognised as insomniac have to be that much more proactive when it comes to stress management, as they suffer from emotional and physiological hyper-arousal that can see stress activate the HPA axis pretty much 24/7. In other words, they are *on*, day and night.

Hyper-aroused people find it hard to unwind, struggle with stressful challenges, or simply stress out when others don't. They tend to internalise negative emotions, which in turn makes them more tense and stressed. They can be irritable and, not surprisingly (given poor sleep and chaotic body chemicals), can fly off the handle at the tiniest provocation.

I can see now that I have a tendency to become hyper-aroused sometimes: over-reactive, but both in a positive, excited, energised way, as well as in a negative, this-is-a-major-problem (when it's not, or doesn't have to be) way. Often it's the result of having loaded too many things on to my to-do list. By the time I realise what's going on, when it's a negative reaction, I can feel the rising tension in my chest, neck, shoulders and face. Frown in place. So I stop, take a deep breath and talk myself down by looking at the trigger from a different point of view.

Emotional stress quickly becomes physiological (which comes down to your health and the biochemistry of emotions, where thoughts and words impact your body chemically, physically and behaviourally). This means that holding on to negative thoughts, reliving stressful events in your mind, or constantly worrying about the possibility of not being able to fall asleep can fast transform into a physical reaction of anxiety, nausea, fear and tension, activating your fight-or-flight response team and its action hormones. Plus, researchers have found that being hyper-aroused leaves insomniacs with a greater (i.e. overactive) whole-brain metabolism, which is unhelpful at night, as this gets in the way of the deactivation of those structures that are keeping us awake.

The secret life of your brain

Scientists have a fair amount of brain kit to play with these days to try to work out what's going on when we're awake and when we're asleep: they have electroencephalogram (EEG) sensors that are attached to the scalp to measure brainwaves, the electrical impulses that see brain cells firing together in a particular rhythm; CAT scans, to take 3D X-ray images of the brain; PET scans that allow us to follow the movement of liquids that have been swallowed; magnetic resonance imaging (MRI) that give detailed images of the brain; and functional MRI (fMRI), which combines detailed images with the ability to track brain activity through blood flow.

It was thanks to the tracking of dyed brain/spinal fluid (cerebrospinal fluid or CSF) as it made its way round the brains and spinal cords of mice that scientists discovered that the brain has a drainage system (the glymphatic system), which only wakes up once we're asleep to give the brain a good scrub down. The spaces between the brain cells were spotted expanding by a dramatic 60 per cent, clearing the way for brain fluids to flush out the brain and carry off any toxic waste that had built up during the day. Stop the glymphatic system from doing its job properly, by not getting enough sleep, and, some scientists believe, you risk Alzheimer's by not giving your brain enough time to rid itself of the toxic molecule build-up (in particular the toxic protein beta- amyloid) that's linked to such neurodegenerative disorders.

What's also been detected is that an exhausted brain starts to eat itself. The 'housekeeping' astrocyte and microglial cells in mice, responsible for clearing out worn-out cells and trimming synapses, go into overdrive when mice are sleep deprived, over-pruning left and right – activity that has again been linked to neurodegeneration and Alzheimer's. Good reasons, if ever you need them, to try to give yourself some quality sleep.

The deeper you go

Brain-testing equipment also shows that we sleep in cycles of roughly 90-minute chunks (anything from 70 to 120 minutes). Not a solid mass of sleep, as was sometimes thought, but one where we repeatedly shift between light sleep and deep sleep and occasionally surface between the two.

Over the course of the 90 minutes, the brain works through various stages of sleep. There are several ways of looking at this, but one is that there are three progressively light-to-deep stages (non-REM/NREM = non-rapid eye movement) and one light dream sleep stage (REM = rapid eye movement). We move between waking, N1, N2, N3 and REM – with N3 being the deepest sleep. And then, with one cycle complete, it starts all over again.

During the day our brainwaves can be super-fast – known as gamma waves – if we're using our brains to learn and to process information. Next, and not so fast, are our beta waves, when we're focused and concentrated, as at work, followed by alpha (relaxed/reflective), theta (drowsy), and, as we subside into rest and finally deep sleep, delta – all of which has been captured by EEG sensors. Our heartbeat, breathing and brainwaves slow down, our muscles get progressively more relaxed, body temperature drops and eye movement slows and stops, ending in a deep, slow-wave sleep that's crucial if we're going to wake up feeling revitalised.

REM, or active sleep, on the other hand, is when most dreams take place, and we get more of this as morning approaches (and more deep sleep in the earlier part of the night). During REM sleep, your blood pressure, heartbeat and breathing rates increase – and chemicals are released so that you are semi-paralysed and don't act out your dreams.

Ideally, the average adult needs seven to eight hours sleep a night for optimal health, depending on the length of their sleep cycle. And it's these cycles that we need to count, rather than the hours we've spent asleep, if we want to wake refreshed at the end of one cycle, instead of groggy because the alarm has woken us up in the middle of a deep sleep.

Five sleep cycles at *circa (c.)* 90 minutes a go will give you roughly 7½ hours of sleep: perfect according to the latest findings. So, for example, if I want to wake up at 7am, I count back five cycles, and the time I'll need to be asleep by is 11.30pm.

The other useful and reassuring thing about knowing you sleep in *c.*90-minute chunks is that you don't have to worry if you momentarily surface between the shallow end of one cycle and the beginning of the next, in the middle of the night. This is not something you need to grab on to in panic as 'broken sleep'. You can relax. Breathe deep. And keep your brainwaves slow. Your body clock and chemicals are primed for sleep, and you can simply move into the next cycle. Wake too early with enough time for another chunk, and you can give it to yourself in the knowledge that you're not going to be forced awake by the alarm during the last part of the cycle filled with dreams as morning approaches, which is something we all want to avoid, because we need those dreams to process our memories, examine problems when we're in a non-emotional state, improve our creativity and lateral thinking skills, and more.

Mixing and mingling

Parasomnias, a rare group of disruptive sleep disorders that take place around sleep, and other more extreme sleep conditions, sit in the muddy waters between being awake and asleep. They take place when the brain moves between deep sleep, dream sleep and wakefulness, where sometimes our dreams can spill over into our conscious world, creating intensely realistic hallucinations. Spill-overs that happen in the morning, as we're coming to, are called hypnopompic, whereas those that take hold as we're going to sleep are hypnogogic.

Sleepwalkers can get dressed, drive, cook – all complex behaviours – with their eyes wide open, but still be in a state of deep sleep. Some people sleep-talk while others can wake up to find the leftovers of a midnight feast in their bed, the messy evidence of their sleep-related eating disorder – raw chicken and a slab of butter being actual examples of what people have found in their bed come morning. Narcoleptics can move suddenly between being awake and asleep at inappropriate times with little barrier between the two. Those suffering from cataplexy, brought on by intense emotions or laughter, lose the use of their muscles when wide awake (just as everyone does during dream sleep, to stop us thrashing about and acting out our dreams), making them collapse on the spot. Sleepers with REM sleep behaviour disorder (RBD), on the other hand, *do* act out their aggressive dreams, usually while still in bed, which is unnerving and sometimes even dangerous for anyone sharing a bed with them. Then there's homicidal sleepwalking and sexsomnia, which both speak for themselves.

For the vast majority, these disorders are just words on a page and nothing to worry about. But what all these night-time and sleep-related antics show is that there is no rock-solid line between being awake and being asleep, which blurs our perception of what is asleep and what is awake. It's even possible for different parts of the brain to be awake and asleep at the same time, which helps to explain why those who have a time of it, trying to wrap themselves in a comforting blanket of deep sleep, might feel as if they've barely slept at all but have hovered in an annoying half-way house, when in fact they *have* slept, at some level.

It all comes down to what we're conscious of, and what we're not conscious of. As Coué put it when writing about sleepwalkers, 'Everyone knows that the somnambulist gets up at night *without waking*, leaves his room after either dressing himself or not, goes downstairs, walks along corridors and, after having executed certain acts or accomplished certain work, returns to his room, goes to bed again, and shows next day the greatest astonishment at finding work finished which he had left unfinished the day before. It is however he himself who has done it without being aware of it. What force has his body obeyed if it is not an unconscious force, in fact his unconscious self?'

While most of the more extreme sleep disorders out there are rare and something that should be handed over to a professional sleep clinic, if necessary, they all take the lid off the fact that being awake and asleep are not, as experts previously thought, two totally separate states of consciousness, but ones that can easily mix and mingle.

One of my big takeaways from all of this has been that I no longer stress out if I feel like I'm only half asleep at night. I tell myself, 'You're getting more sleep than you realise', and 'There isn't a hard line between deep rest and sleep, the conscious and the unconscious,' and I find this reassuring and calming, to the extent that any niggling insomnia panic immediately backs down and I can relax into sleep and leave my conscious mind behind. This knowledge used to help me when I was struggling to go to sleep, and it can still help me to stop worrying and to move away from semi-awake sleep into a deep, quality sleep if I wake in the middle of the night.

To nap or not to nap

Naps can be a lifesaver. For those who prefer a mini reboot during the day, rather than seven-plus hours at night, or are sleep short for whatever reason, a productive power nap is the way to go, whether it's a quick 15 to 20-minute top-up, a longer 26-minute NASA nap (see page 54), or a *c.*90-minute full reboot. (Not that I nap, unless ill, but I know plenty of people who rely on them.) Today a 15 to 20-minute nap, sometimes called a stage 2 nap, is often put forward as the ideal booster – the argument being that any more snoozing than this risks you getting into a deep sleep, which can be hard to break out of.

The NASA nap

NASA first argued the case for strategic naps back in 1995, when its researchers argued that a 26-minute mid-flight nap dramatically improved the safety and performance of tired pilots.

A popular tip for keeping naps short is to grab a cup of caffeinated tea or coffee during the sleep zone of 1 until 3pm, when our body clocks take an energy dip, then go for a nap and let the caffeine act as an alarm clock when it starts to kick in $c.$30 minutes later (although the earlier the better, so there's less caffeine in your system come bedtime). Napping after 3pm is not a good idea, as this is getting too close to your evening wind-down and will throw off your 24-hour sleep–wake rhythm, just as babies' daytime naps need to be restricted to earlier in the day if parents want them to sleep well at night.

We all have a natural up/down daily energy flow, which explains why 1 until 3pm is the prime time for naps. For the majority, our brains are sharpest in the morning, making this the ideal time to tackle the most challenging to-dos, then they are on a gentle decline after lunch, with a real dip around 3pm, after which our energy levels creep back up to a $c.$6pm peak.

If your sleep debt is huge, however, a bite-sized power nap won't cut it. Your mind is likely to shut down any chance it gets for a daytime catch-up, and if you're that sleep deprived, your body is crying out for a full sleep cycle to claw back some urgently needed sleep. For those who are cognitively struggling, unable to focus effectively, a 60–90-minute nap that ends before 3pm, so as not to interfere with the coming night's sleep, is said to be as good as a full night's sleep when it comes to learning. This means it can give your brain a real lift, whatever you're doing, so it's worth considering if you're really short on sleep and can work this into your day.

From gamma to beta, alpha, theta and delta

We can switch down a gear from beta to alpha during the day simply by taking a break to rest or go for a stroll, or by giving ourselves five minutes to mull something over. Shutting your eyes intensifies alpha by blocking out visual stimulations, so just allowing yourself to unwind and close your eyes in bed at night already puts you on the road to alpha and theta. Breathe deeply and imagine your brainwaves slowing down, and this helps too, as a biology-based sleep suggestion, something that can be used when you go to bed or if you wake in the middle of the night. I do this fairly often and am always reassured by how effective it is – visualising my brainwaves changing from being fast, dense, compressed and spiky to being more relaxed, slow, rounded, spaced out and lolloping along, moving into sleep.

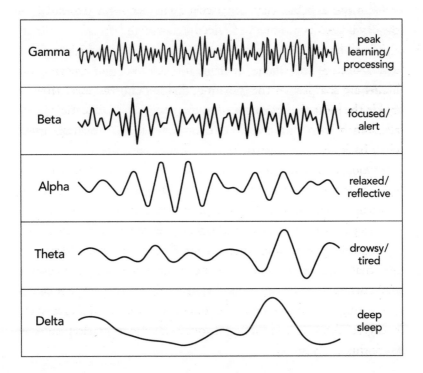

Theta brainwaves can also be activated during the day when you're day-dreaming, on autopilot, doing a job or task that you don't have to think about (such as walking a well-trodden route), or meditating. If you're having trouble settling your mind for sleep, or you have woken in the night and want to sink back into sleep, a few minutes of deep breathing or meditation (gently focusing on the breath) can help to activate your theta waves, and from there it's one step back to delta (deep sleep).

When you take a look at sleep history, it's clear that surfacing from sleep in the middle of the night is nothing to fixate on. Historian Roger Ekirch's seminal book *At Day's Close: A History of Nighttime* delves into the history of sleep and concludes that two sleeps were the norm in pre-industrial Western Europe, when evenings were not made use of as they are today. Many people went to bed early to conserve energy, stay warm and safe, and save on food and fire, and an hour or two of 'quiet wakefulness' in the middle of the night was an accepted part of life.

Humans, it appears, would go to bed early, sleep for one chunk of time and then either lie in bed relaxing, rested and dreamy, ruminating or thinking over their dreams, having sex, chatting, drifting in a semi-conscious state likened to meditation, or sometimes get up to do something useful, visit a neighbour or do some chores, before settling down for their second sleep of the night.

Our shift away from two sleeps to one came with scientific progress and a rejection of the superstition that night-time is filled with danger, evil spirits, disease, ghosts, hellish fear, and malevolent witches, pixies and trolls, argues Ekirch, together with the elongation of day into night with affordable candles, oil lamps and electricity. But that doesn't mean that this biphasic sleep pattern that was once standard won't surface from time to time. If it does, our best bet is to try to relax, enjoy the silence and the opportunity to rest and reflect, as our ancestors used to do and accept the blurred boundary between being awake and asleep. With what you know about sleep biology and your imagination on board, you can just let your sleep-inducing neurons take over.

Simply being aware is all that you need

You only need to have an awareness of this sleep biology and how the body works. It's not necessary to remember every little detail or biological name. When I sat in on Professor Whorwell and Dr Hasan's sessions with their patients, they gave just an outline of the biology involved and what changes were needed for the body to run smoothly.

In the biology-based sleep suggestions I give myself, or the direct action I take to help things along, it's enough to know and remind myself that bright daylight and darkness at night are activating the chemicals and biological rhythms that are essential for my sleep–wake cycle. I'm aware of this as I load my mornings with light and dim my nights. Furthermore, I know that deep breathing at night dramatically slows down my brainwaves, as well as setting up the rest-and-digest state I need to be in to sleep. It does this via the vagus nerve (a nerve that connects the digestive system with the brain), which carries a slow-down message all around my body that I can visualise.

Stress, hyper-arousal and overstimulation disrupt sleep through all that excess cortisol, but there's much that I can do to counteract this, both during the day and last thing at night – not least, by consciously and proactively cutting my stress chemicals while boosting the four happy hormones, or by changing my perception of immediate stressors (see Chapter 6).

I know that staring into a pitch-dark bedroom will produce melatonin and GABA, which will help to turn off my awake state, and that there's a flip-flop sleep switch that I can help activate by strengthening the hand of my sleep-inducing neurons, which I imagine piled high on an old-fashioned set of scales until the sleep-inducing side is so high and heavy that it drops down low enough to trigger the switch.

By sticking out my extremities – hands and feet – from under the duvet, I will bring down my core temperature, which is needed for sleep and is useful if I wake from overheating in the middle of the night. By being aware that we sleep in roughly 90-minute chunks, I can build my night around this and go back to sleep for another chunk if I wake too early. Telling myself that my sleep drive/pressure is gathering chemical momentum helps me to stop overriding it or pushing through exhaustion rather than going to bed when tired. Simply running through some of this in my mind last thing at night has a real physiological effect; for example, I might remind myself that my GABA and melatonin levels are high and rising, that my sleep drive is strong and that slow, deep breathing is moving my brainwaves from beta to alpha, while I tell myself, 'I am going to sleep now'.

Bringing all this together with light, habit and food science, plus day-to-day suggestions, all considered in relation to sleep, I can now not only support my natural sleep–wake cycle and my in-built sleep drive but I can also systematically strengthen them so that it's inevitable that I sleep soundly.

---

4 top tips

1. Work with your sleep drive throughout your day.
2. Take a 26-minute NASA nap, or a c.90-minute full reboot early in the day, if needed.
3. Remind yourself that the flip-flop switch will put you to sleep.
4. Breathe deeply to slow brainwaves down – you can also visualise this.

Chapter 3

The Big Primordial Tick-Tock

From north London to Oregon's Mount Hood,
we need to light-grab morning, noon and night to
choreograph our day.

Outside it was dark, cold and raining while I was sitting in a crowded north London crypt with a view of tombstones, listening to Professor Steve Jones talk about his book *Here Comes the Sun*. I hadn't realised the jaw-dropping, negative health repercussions of too little sun before this evening, with vitamin D so vital for us to stay healthy and to stop our bones bending from rickets, but I *was* very aware of how daylight-deficient most of us are and how this is impacting our sleep.

I had followed a silent stream of umbrellad figures to find the entrance to the crypt, tucked away down the side of its church, which was a welcome beacon of light on a bitter January night. Later, splashing back through the rain as I left, in what was an almost pitch-black graveyard, it struck me how rarely urban life is plunged into such a rich and soothing darkness.

You wouldn't think anyone could be light deprived in this

post-industrial, electric-light-saturated world, but ironically our natural *c.*24-hour sleep–wake cycle has been turned upside down by dim indoor mornings and brighter-than-natural nights – leaving our bodies starved of daylight, and of the darkness of night, too. The upshot of this artificially lit world in which we find ourselves is that the light–dark messages bombarding our brains are all wrong, leaving our body clocks in chaos and our sleep–wake cycle more than a little confused.

With around 90 per cent of our time now spent indoors, rather than tilling the land, it stands to reason that our daylight hours are darker than they used to be. That might sound counter-intuitive, given the level of artificial light indoors, but the fact is that the electric light we live by is no match for the daylight outside, even on a cloudy day. To confound our brains even further, our nights are lighter than they ever have been, filled with street lights, house lights and screens with their blue–white light that we hold up close – nice and bright.

But our sleep–wake cycle can't function properly like this. As we saw in the previous chapter, humans are programmed to sleep when it's dark and wake when it's light, using light cues to synchronise our body clocks (our circadian clocks) to the 24-hour day – a dark–light cycle that's the result of the Earth circling around the sun. What our bodies are primed to do, day in, day out, is track and fall in line with the Earth's rotation using the rising and setting of the sun to keep every cell synced and running smoothly. To do this, our eyes scan the light around us, which sends messages to the hypothalamus in our brain, and the brain takes action accordingly, either releasing the sleepy hormone melatonin at night, or suppressing it during the day. What's more, our bodies are only *roughly* in line with the 24-hour clock outside (running to 24 hours and 11 minutes on average), so we need to be constantly re-set, using daylight and night darkness as our markers. This was not a problem for thousands of years until the arrival of the electric light some 140 years ago, but it's a very big problem now.

From outer space to you

NASA has long studied the effects of light on its pilots, who are exposed to a sunrise and a sunset every 90 minutes as they move around Earth in orbit (a 90-minute day, rather than the 24-hour day the rest of us get). The space agency is at the forefront of light science, looking into how indoor lighting can mirror the 24-hour sky light and tackle sleep disorders head-on to overcome chronic sleep loss or circadian misalignment, not only for astronauts but also for sleep-deprived populations as a whole.

'Astronauts living in outer space during space travel have a number of health issues, but one of them is problems with disruption of the circadian system and disruption of sleep,' NASA light scientist, George C. Brainard, tells me. It was his team who first predicted that there must be undiscovered photoreceptors in the eye that react to light.

'The circadian system regulates virtually every tissue system in the body,' continues Dr Brainard, who has directed Jefferson University's Light Research Program since 1984, 'and when you disrupt it and dysregulate long term, there are long-term health consequences associated with that. Everything from increased cancer risk, heart disease, GI dysfunction, metabolic disorders and so forth, so it's not a trivial thing.'

Seventy-one per cent of the astronauts on Space Shuttle and 75 per cent on the International Space Station (ISS) are reliant on sleep-promoting drugs, but they still report sub-standard sleep (just under six hours on the Shuttle), in what is a high-risk job. Brainard and his team were therefore called on to install a state-of-the-art lighting system on the United States portion of the ISS in 2018, modulated over 24 hours 'to give the astronauts a better visual environment and to improve circadian regulation and improve sleep'.

Also, thanks to the discovery of that unknown photoreceptor (photosensitive retinal ganglion cells), scientists now know that there are two levels of activity going on in the eye: the conscious experience of vision and what we see, and the unconscious control our eyes have over our behaviour and physiology, including our body's circadian clocks and our sleep–wake cycle.

What Brainard and his team really wanted to pinpoint, however, was that if white light wakes us up, by making the pineal gland suppress sleep-inducing melatonin, what about all the other wavelengths – from short-wavelength light (violet, indigo and blue), to middle wavelengths (green and yellow) and longer wavelengths (orange and red)? To answer this, tests were carried out over seven years on behalf of the National Space Biomedical Research Institute to see how the eye and the pineal gland would react to different coloured lights and the effect these different wavelengths have on our melatonin levels.

'What we found was that different wavelengths had different potencies for regulating melatonin,' says Brainard, 'but those wavelengths in the short wavelength end of the spectrum, specifically in the blue-appearing part of the spectrum [all bright white lights contain blue] could elicit a strong melatonin suppression.' And with this wavelength, you get a 'very powerful suppression with very, very little light energy'. Meaning a short blast of the blue light you get on your mobile phone will knock melatonin production on the head, whereas longer wavelengths (orange and red) will not suppress melatonin, allowing levels to rise and fall as you need them to.

The long goodnight

Our bedtime routine needs to start the moment we wake up by opening our curtains/black-out blinds to let the daylight pour in. This not only helps to reset our body clocks by lining us up with the 24-hour, night–day light clock outside, but it also shoos the remaining melatonin away and kick-starts our body's natural sleep countdown: that sleep drive/pressure that builds up the longer we're awake, making us increasingly tired as night draws in.

Light and dark have to structure our day. For optimum sleep that's natural and effortless, we need to get outside, sit by a window, take in the sky and bask in the light of day, and night, to register or recreate (using a light box or light blockers, if necessary) the natural light signals that go with the rising and the setting of the sun.

Our mornings in particular need to be loaded with as much daylight as we can manage to support our 24-hour biological rhythms. We need to light-grab, as the day goes on, at any chance we can get or can orchestrate, making a point to look up at the sky for the full force of that light. As night descends, our body responds to dusk and darkness to get ready for sleep, whether we step outside or recreate it by reaching for dimmer switches, candles or black-out blinds. Whatever the time of day, our bodies are hardwired to tune in with the light outside, or whatever is around us. And the photoreceptors in our eyes are ready and waiting to set off chemical cascades that either keep us awake or prepare us for sleep.

All is one, and one is all

Plants know when to open and close their petals, birds when to migrate and humans when to wake and sleep, all thanks to internal rhythms that work in sync with natural light and surrounding temperature to keep a whole number of activities running to timetable. We don't just *respond* to rays of light streaming in in the morning – our body *anticipates* them. It knows where it is in the night–day cycle and is ready, biologically, with a rising body temperature and the release of action hormones a good hour before we wake and well before the alarm kicks off.

It's strange to think that we're full of tiny body clocks, so to speak, but every cell in the body is in on the act. We're not alone in this, given that all organisms have circadian clocks at a molecular level, it's just that in humans there's also a master clock in the brain's hypothalamus (the suprachiasmatic nucleus – SCN) that's trying to make everything keep time. And it's the SCN that's officially in charge of our sleep–wake cycle.

Not only do we need to line up the SCN with the 24-hour light clock and temperature outside but we also need to make sure that *all* the clocks in our body are working as one, if we want to get the best sleep possible. While the SCN is controlled by light, the peripheral clocks in our body's organs are largely controlled by what and when we eat, or when we fast (that gap between dinner/a late-night snack and breakfast). Any erratic eating habits we might have will ensure that our light and food clocks are not keeping the same time, and this is something that needs to be sorted if our body has any hope of being in tune with itself, with internal clocks harmonised and biological oscillations working in tandem.

Although it might seem odd that adults need to be deliberately tuned in to night and day, just as newborn babies are taught to sleep when it's dark and wake when it's light, the body's natural sleep drive that builds up during the day is not only being skewed by artificial light but by the fact that many people work late, party late, watch television in bed and check social media well after lights-out – all stimulants that disrupt our circadian clocks. Add to this a high-fat, high-calorie Western diet (which also messes with our sleep – see Chapter 7), late evening meals or snacking heavily right up until bedtime, and you have the central body clock that's controlling the body's sleep–wake cycle at odds with the body's feeding rhythms, which is a recipe for sleep disaster.

Primed time

A controlled sleep-lab study by a team of researchers in Germany, led by Professor Jan Born, found that our body starts getting ready to wake up a good hour before we get up (c.90 minutes), slowly releasing the action hormones we need to surface into the day. What's particularly interesting is that sleepers in the study who were told they would be woken up at 6am, were alert and ready to start their day at this time, whereas others, who were tricked into thinking that they could sleep until 9am, but in fact were hauled out of bed at 6am, were groggy and not remotely ready; their bodies and action hormones were clearly banking on having a lie-in, thanks to the suggestion that they had been given.

Blinking into the sunlight

On the back of all this newfound light knowledge, I bought myself a new gadget: a hand-held light meter. It's not something that might set many a pulse racing, but it's fascinating to me, nonetheless, to be able to activate it on my desk at different times of the day, or on the kitchen table, in the garden, or the street out front, to see what I'm working with inside compared to the great outdoors. And I was taken aback from day one to discover just how dark and gloomy my largely desk-bound, indoor life can be.

The light around us is measured in lux, with a reasonably well-lit room giving you around 300 lux and bright office lighting going up to *c.*500 lux. But step outside for a minute and this jumps up to 1,000 lux on an overcast day, 10,000–25,000 lux in full daylight and 100,000 lux in direct sunlight. No competition.

While I knew that my study wasn't the brightest indoor space, I didn't expect it to be *that* dark, but the reading I got from my desk was just *c.*100 lux, coaxed up to a little over 300 when placed directly under my desk lamp. Outside, even on a cloudy-but-bright day, the garden table pulls in 6,000–7,000 lux, and can bask in 87,000-plus lux at mid UK summer.

The benefits of a light box

I've now installed a light box (10,000 lux) on my desk to give my room some extra oomph and to anchor my body clocks in something equivalent to that early morning light that's happening outside. I do also make a point of taking in the sky throughout the day for some full-force daylight and for my master body clock to register the time of day and sync with that. (I never look directly at the sun, of course, as this causes UV-induced eye damage to the retinas.)

A light box is also good for waking us up, boosting our focus and alertness, prompting our body to produce less day-time melatonin and more mood-enhancing serotonin, especially during those grey winter months when we're not getting much sun. It is for this reason that light boxes are championed for those who suffer from seasonal affective disorder (SAD). We do also need actual sun, when possible, for vitamin D, particularly given that a vitamin-D deficiency is linked to insomnia. As far as sleep is concerned, however, you need to absorb that beam of blue light as early as possible in the day (these shorter wavelengths also penetrate our skin), and far away from your nights so that it doesn't confuse the light–brain signals you need to take in and, in the process, prevent your sleep drive from cranking up as the day moves forward.

In search of darkness

It's light, or rather the lack of it, that we really need to embrace towards the end of our day to help us sleep more easily, as this is the main external trigger – or zeitgeber – our bodies rely on to get our pre-bed chemical preparations underway. As darkness closes in, our pineal gland wakes up and releases sleepy melatonin into the blood, while the hypothalamus unleashes the inhibitory amino acid GABA to close down our awake state.

Melatonin levels start inching up when it gets dark, and will stay in our systems throughout the night, peaking at around 2–4am before subsiding as light filters in at dawn, and finally tapering off at around 9am. By removing brighter-than-bright lights from our evenings and then staring into the darkness of a pitch-black bedroom after lights-out, we can help this process along, boosting both melatonin and GABA, because the message to our brain will be clear: it's dark, it's night, it's time to prepare for sleep and time for our core body temperature to drop, which we also need in order to go to sleep and to stay asleep, with the ideal room temperature for this being 17°C/62.6F°.

Bright lights, in contrast to dark, stifle melatonin and GABA but improve our mood and increase our serotonin levels. They are perfect if we are feeling down, or climbing out of bed ready to tackle the day, but they are a circadian-clock setback if it's time to sleep. This is why we need to weight our mornings with light and turn down the dimmer switch on our evenings, to give our circadian clocks the signals and synchronicity they need. Even some who are blind can make use of these light or dark triggers to line up their body clocks with the day and night going on outside, thanks to those photoreceptors in our eyes that respond to light, not sight, to line us up with the 24-hour clock.

Shaded from the glare

Melatonin not only helps us sleep, it also boosts our immune system, and is a powerful antioxidant and an oncostatic hormone (which halts the spread of cancer), making our exposure to too much light at night a serious health problem that shouldn't be ignored, and our melatonin levels something we need to guard. Just driving across town at night can expose us to the dangers of light pollution, thanks to the increasing use of energy-efficient, blue-rich LED lighting, which suppresses melatonin and more, according to the American Medical Association (AMA). Humans, birds and other creatures are struggling with sleep, migration and all sorts, thanks to this excess light at night. With a third of the global population no longer able to see the Milky Way due to light pollution, the growth of international dark-sky parks is just one of the initiatives fighting back against this encroachment on our nights.

Light at night is also pushing society towards obesity, with countless studies making the link between our longer days, brighter nights, disrupted metabolism, circadian clocks and feeding rhythms, and society's growing weight problem. One study, for example, found that mice housed in a bright-light–dim-light space that was never dark, put on significantly more weight than mice fed the same diet on a standard light–dark cycle. The light-drenched mice were also less able to tolerate glucose, which left them with more glucose in their blood (a precursor to diabetes) – plus they ate more of their quota of food during the light phase than their counterparts did.

Global obesity has almost tripled since 1975, with most people living in countries where obesity is more of a killer than being underweight, according to the World Health Organization (WHO).

Light, food consumption, metabolism and the body's circadian clocks are all intertwined: the light in your life and the timing of what you eat can make you fatter, or if you turn it round the other way – with plenty of dark to balance the light – it can help you lose weight.

Humans are particularly sensitive to the blue–white light emitted by high-intensity LEDs, as is our melatonin off-button. White LED lamp lights 'have five times greater impact on circadian sleep rhythms than conventional street lamps', warns the AMA, which is urging communities to use 'the lowest emission of blue light possible to reduce glare', for driver safety. The AMA also believes that we should shield LED lights and dim them at low-peak periods, to protect our own melatonin levels, and to stop unsettling the rhythms of the environment and animals from a light that's too much at odds with the real night and day.

Night-shift workers, not surprisingly, take a big hit when it comes to sleep-related illnesses, caused by erratic hours and erratic dark and light signals: disrupted sleep; excessive exposure to artificial light at night (ALAN); and low levels of melatonin, which is linked to cancer (in particular prostate and breast cancer); diabetes, cardiovascular risks and obesity (tests exposing chicks to light showed that the more light they lived by, the heavier the chicks); mood disorders and age-related macular degeneration.

A study of French pastry chefs and shopkeepers found that their early shift-work schedules put them at high risk of developing sleep disorders (although napping was put forward as an effective countermeasure to this). Not that these sleep-related health risks can be ignored by anyone in today's 24/7 gig economy, where nine-to-five office hours are a thing of the past for many and an estimated 75 per cent of the workforce in industrialised societies is said to have worked shifts or at night at some point.

WHO has declared shift work to be a risk factor for cancer, and although research into the best counter-measures to adopt is limited, better sleep, together with a healthy diet and exercise, is widely recommended.

It seems that night-shift workers could also benefit from making their 'days' as bright as possible, and their 'evenings' and 'nights' as dusk-like and dark as possible. This would go some way in giving their bodies the light–dark balance that we all need, while increasing their melatonin and GABA levels when they're ready to go to sleep, and it would give their immune systems a boost. Studies suggest that shielding yourself from natural light at the end of a night shift will improve the quality of your sleep. For everyone else, in contrast, softer, shaded night light is something to be prized and protected.

What time zones are you in?

It's little wonder that our body clocks can get so misaligned, given the pace of life these days, which has taken off since electricity opened up our nights and airplanes gave us the ability to travel much further and faster. In the past, we travelled more slowly, as Coué did when he travelled by boat to North America, which gave our bodies ample time to adjust. In addition, we couldn't use our evenings as we do now – candles hadn't been made cheap enough for all and street lamps were yet to light up our cities, making a night life a safe, viable option. And even when evening light became more widespread, the light that was on offer was soft, warm and circadian-friendly.

Today, our bodies are often left disgruntled and out of sync, and our sleep–wake cycle disjointed by jet lag or social jet lag – its stay-at-home mini-me. Whether we hop from one time zone to another, with our body playing catch-up, or we switch from midweek 'school-night' hours to social-animal hours at the weekend, both wreak havoc with our body's efforts to buddy up with the Earth's rotation in relation to the sun.

Social jet lag can, of course, be minimised with as regular wake-up and go-to-bed times as we can manage around the work and social life that we need or want to have. But any jet lag can leave us with acute short-term sleep disruption that can become a long-term problem if left to dig in. (It's thought that the jet lag we get from travelling west to east is worse than that from east to west, because it's easier for us to delay our body clocks than to advance them.)

Once I would have been reaching for prescription sleeping pills to avoid losing my mind from lack of sleep due to long-haul jet lag after flying back to the UK from visiting in-laws in West Coast America. Now, however, I find it's enough to get as much exposure as possible to daylight after touchdown and to keep dousing my mornings with maximum daylight on subsequent days. And I combine this with re-structuring my day around breakfast, lunch and dinner in line with the new time zone I'm in, together with other sleep-friendly habits that I automatically lock into.

A spotlight into your brain

Away from spaceflights, night work and street lights, the biggest sleep-disrupters and blue-light-polluting culprits are, of course, smartphones, tablets, computers and large flat-screen TVs: an intense wrap-around of LEDs that didn't exist a decade ago and is now befuddling our circadian clocks and sparking a dramatic increase in sleep deprivation and chronic sleep disorders.

Our need to connect, just one more time, before the lights go out, and perhaps once more after that, and after that ... is tipping over into compulsive behaviour for some of us and blasting our eyes with bright, midday light when they should be soaking in a black, star-spangled sky or a blacked-out, go-to-sleep room. Blue-light-blocking glasses (with orange-red tinted lenses), computer filters, screen dusks (f.lux.com) and warm-light apps, go some way to offset this stay-awake screen glut; however, what we really need to do to neutralise this LED excess and, crucially, the mentally engaging, over-stimulating communication overload that goes with it, is to shut it all down and give ourselves the recommended 90 minutes of dim or red-spectrum surround lighting before we want to go to sleep. This will not only allow our melatonin levels to rise but will also stop us from being over-stimulated and hyper-aroused just before bed.

Phones are possibly the biggest offender when it comes to ruining our sleep, due to our inability to put them to bed at night. In the UK, the number of people watching TV, checking emails or using laptops/gadgets just before bed has actually declined slightly in recent years, according to The Great British Bedtime Report. Nevertheless, 38 per cent of adults say that they keep a smartphone in their bedroom, and 57 per cent of children say they sleep with their phone next to them at night, according to a report by Childwise. Problematic phone use among young adults is said to be higher in the UK, France and Belgium, compared with Poland and Germany, for example, while 60 per cent of Belgians, aged 18–94, were found to take their phone into their bedroom overnight.

Seventy-one per cent of Americans say that they have their phones in their bedroom every night. Three per cent actually hold their phones in bed at night, while only 4 per cent have no idea where their phone is when they tuck themselves in. Outside the bedroom, the National Sleep Foundation found that 90 per cent of Americans use their gadgets in the last hour before bed, and a plethora of surveys show that teenagers use mobile phones up to and right through the night, which has a negative impact on their sleep, daytime energy, stress and anxiety levels, and ability to focus.

'If somebody gets up and pulls over their cell phone to stare at it and they see an interesting email, or they're unable to sleep and they pick up a video, or a game, or whatever,' says Brainard, 'they're actually delivering a stimulus that is potentially alerting, defeating their chance to go back to sleep.' Anything more than a few minutes on a mobile phone at night will give you a strong glare of blue LED light, right into the receptor in your eyes, suppressing melatonin and upsetting your sleep, as LEDs 'emit very strongly right in that part of the spectrum that the eye is most sensitive to, for regulating melatonin, circadian rhythms and neural behavioural responses,' he adds. And our receptors are more sensitive during the evening and night. That's to say that if you wake in the night and reach for a screen, it's game over. You're telling your brain it's time to engage and wake up. And it will.

If you're a social-media junkie struggling to sleep, the advice is: turn everything off. Get screens out of your bedroom. Give yourself some offline/out-of-office hours. And if you can't cut the mobile phone umbilical cord and ban it from your bedroom, you can always switch it to silent mode and turn it face down – to stop those through-the-night missives tempting you out of bed and snapping you awake.

TVs are not considered to be so bad, depending on your level of engagement. They're not right in your face, for one. And for some they act as the perfect sleeping pill, unless you're a binge-viewer. Binge viewers have more chance of suffering from poorer sleep quality, greater fatigue and insomnia symptoms, according to research. The argument being that we're more likely to feel the pull to binge view when programmes have lots of interconnecting storylines from episode to episode, designed to keep us hooked. This then leaves us with 'cognitive pre-sleep arousal' (that is, an overstimulated mind, stuffed with plotlines and drama) just before bed, which we'll need time to unwind from, and which will, obviously, delay us from falling asleep. And if you think it's a great idea to watch a nail-biting, anxiety-inducing, action-packed film just before bed, stand back and watch your adrenaline and cortisol levels run riot, shoving melatonin and your rest-and-digest system to one side, as this shift in hormones makes it harder for you to relax, switch off and go to sleep, as well as disrupting the quality of your night's sleep.

Domestic sunsets – and the polar opposite

It's far too easy to miss both sunrise and sunset if you live in an urban or built-up setting with only tantalising glimpses here and there, but we can still help to keep our molecularly circadian clocks happy with a bit of dusk simulation, which at least sends the right evening-light signals in the direction of our brain.

I turn down the lights in my children's rooms a good hour before they go to bed. Hall lights go off. And, for myself, I turn down everything from around 9pm onwards: warm display lights start softening my screens from 7pm, computer shut-down is around 9.30pm, and I use the lowest light possible in my bedroom and bathroom so that nothing gets in the way of that sleep drive and those mounting melatonin and GABA levels. Even when friends are round, and evenings that much later, lights are dimmed as the evening progresses.

By progressively dimming house lights as evening turns to night, we are, of course, actively helping our circadian rhythm tune in to the night outside, by structuring our day around light and dark. We can also make use of the orange and red bulbs (long wavelength light) that Brainard's team found so helpful with sleep. And by showering ourselves with blue lights in the morning, we're able to tackle the other end of the problem as well.

Tests carried out at the at the Concordia Research Station in

Antarctica (where sunlight is non-existent for four months during winter, creating non-stop darkness that upends circadian rhythms), found that concentrated exposure to blue-enriched white light stopped circadian disruption and sleep loss. Even short bursts of light at the right time of day get quick results, improving sleep and alertness, moods and circadian rhythm, as decades of research have shown. This has led to an upsurge in offices investing in 'daylighting', the development of natural-light solutions to boost productivity. Electrochromic 'smart' office windows have been shown to increase sleep duration by an average of 46 minutes a night (compared with minimal exposure to daylight) and boost cognitive function by 42 per cent. Daylighting ramps up energy levels, productivity and cognitive function to improve well-being and sleep. It is also the reason why giant mirrors were installed to bounce winter sunlight into the sun-deprived Norwegian village of Rjukan.

For those living in northern latitudes, where daylight can be very limited, bright blue-white interior lighting during the day, and particularly in the morning, is clearly the way to go for better sleep (and for better moods, etc.), and could be given additional morning clout with the concentrated 'daylight' that comes from a light box. When there is natural daylight, the best advice would be to soak it up, and around that create those day–night, light–dark cues the best you can.

The future is rosy

Camping on Mount Hood in the wilds of Oregon a few years back, with its icy mountain streams, stratospherically tall fir trees and intensely dark nights, was another of those times that brought home to me how bright urban life tends to be and how unusual and relaxing it is to be submerged in the darkness of night. What I didn't know at the time is that camping is a fast way to sort out our body clocks, whether they're muddled by jet lag or by modern life – syncing us, as it does, with night and day.

Even a short weekend away under the stars in the summer months, equipped with flashlights but offline, can spike melatonin levels that much earlier, bringing sleep forward by nearly two hours, research has found. And a week-long winter camping trip with no artificial light makes campers go to sleep up to 2½ hours earlier than they would at home, with a natural sleep–wake rhythm settling in from *c*.10pm until 6am.

Back home, indoor light can be used in much the same way to mirror the light outdoors, although, of course, this will be less effective if you're not offline. Likewise, keeping an eye on the time during the day can help us to re-align our body clocks, and is something we can run alongside regular sky-watching light-grabs. After all, our brain uses the daily schedule we impose on it to help sync our circadian rhythms, so by checking in regularly ('It's 11am – I'll be going to sleep in about 12 hours') we can further cement the sleep countdown with this time cue and help to reinforce the light–brain feedback loop that keeps everything running as it should.

Cut to the future. Our home's bespoke lighting could be fine-tuned by experts to carry us through the day: from a gentle dawn-breaking glow, to an energy boosting blue light beam, to a soft warm evening, into dusk, a 'don't wake me up it's night-time' rosy bathroom hue and a pitch-black bedroom. For now, there's the effective, affordable and tech-free option that's there for everyone: by using daylight to start your bedtime routine the moment you wake up, you can anchor your body clock by letting natural light flood in. Take breakfast in the brightest spot you can find, get outside, go for a walk, work by a window or outdoors and light-grab as the day goes on. Load your mornings with daylight. Dim your nights, into an orange/red glow, like the soft light of candles, gas lamps and campfires of old before darkness descends, and your circadian clocks will love you for it.

4 top tips

1. Light-grab morning daylight, to sync in with the Earth's rotation and orbit of the sun.
2. Cut bright lights at night, to sleep easy *and* lose weight.
3. Have 90 minutes before sleep free from in-your-face use of phone, tablet or computer screen.
4. Stare into your pitch-dark bedroom at night, to up GABA and melatonin levels.

Chapter 4

A Carrot for Your Habit – How to Create Positives for Sleep

It's all very well being told to turn your bedroom into a
haven, but how does that *really* help?

Émile Coué was front-page news in the 1920s. Everyone from French
farmers to medics, royalty, aristocracy and politicians across Europe
and North America was tripping over themselves to visit him in his
home town of Nancy, or play host to him, or catch him on one of
his sell-out tours. He was mobbed when the transatlantic ship *The
Majestic* docked in New York, and his visit to London in 1921 was
a showstopper. 'The roadway to where he stayed was lined with limousines and perambulators, bath chairs and sick beds,' wrote J. Louis
Orton, once a colleague and co-author, later more of a rival.

As Coué wrote:

It is impossible to think of two things at once. Every thought
entirely filling our mind becomes true for us and tends to transform
itself into action. Every idea that we put into the mind becomes

a reality in so far as it is within the realms of possibility ... Thus you think: I do not sleep at night, and you do not sleep! What is insomnia? It is the idea that when you go to bed, you will not sleep! The person who sleeps well at night is the person who knows very well that in going to bed, he will sleep well!

Thought habits

Now, both Coué and Waters were very focused on our thought habits. Not just the split-second effect thoughts have on the chemical cascades going on inside us, but also their impact on our ongoing emotions, behaviour and health. And they argued that by bringing in new thought habits, layering them up via conscious auto-suggestion, we can cover up our old habits, which lets the new ones reign. 'How is one to explain to oneself and to explain to others that the repetition of the same words "I am going to sleep ... " etc. has the power to produce the effect, and above all so powerful an effect that it is a certain one?' wrote Coué, in a question that he then answered: 'The repetition of the same words forces one to think of them and when we think of them they become true for us and transform themselves into reality.'

Thought habits are only half of the equation, of course, as there are those other behavioural habits that we're all locked into, day in, day out, whether we're aware of them or not, such as a morning routine that we stick to like glue, a route we always take to get to a familiar destination, or having a tendency to procrastinate when faced with a tedious task, or to comfort eat/drink when we're stressed out. Our thought habits do, however, control us far more than we tend to real- ise, as culturally some of our thought habits are so ingrained that they can even improve our cognitive abilities, all based on where we live and how we've been conditioned to think.

In the Western world, for example, we tend to see mental chal- lenges and efforts to resist temptation as draining. Tackle something particularly tough, and we're likely to feel we need a break. In India it's the opposite. Indians, according to research, expect to gather brainpower and mental energy with every challenge they take on, getting sharper and more cognitively focused, no matter how many hours tick by.

In the study 'Reverse ego-depletion: Acts of self-control can improve subsequent performance in Indian cultural contexts', which proved this point, those taking part were dealt one tricky mental task after another. But where the Westerners crashed and burned after the first hurdle, the Indians did even better on their second challenge. Whereas one mindset lamented brain overload, the other powered ahead. Cultural suggestions can be that powerful.

Irrespective of whether your unwanted sleep patterns are triggered by things you habitually think or by things you habitually do, or both, *all* habits are built the same way. And the latest scientific revelations about habits are comforting because they reveal that any habit can be methodically disrupted and replaced. Any one of us can rewire our mind, body and behaviour by dismantling and re-constructing habits from scratch, including the way we think, feel and sleep. We can even tempt our brain to take up a new habit if we offer it a decent enough reward, which is where the 'turn your bedroom into a haven' idea comes in, because, as we'll see later, a bedroom overflowing with positive associations will help a desirable sleep habit stick.

Our autopilot life

One of my worst sleep habits was bedding down for hours and hours of pillow thoughts, which are often blamed for keeping people awake. My mind clearly saw bed as my time to think things through, especially when I hadn't had any downtime during the day. Preoccupations, tomorrow's to-do list, worries, that day's events, work, re-occurring positive or negative thought loops, plot lines and the rest, would take over, engaging my mind, pushing me past exhaustion, overriding my sleep drive and the shut-down chemical messenger GABA, plus the sleepy hormone melatonin, for hours, until insomnia fear (an anxious lurch in the gut) and then insomnia set in.

Just moving off to bed could set off habitual sleep thoughts, tinged with dread, about how long it was going to take me to get to sleep, how little sleep I was likely to get that night, how fed up I was about not being able to sleep. All these thoughts and expectations affecting my body, setting off a chemical reaction that further stymied sleep.

One bad night's sleep doesn't have to be a problem. Even a handful of bad nights and you're probably still OK, if a bit wired and feeling the strain. But once those sleepless nights start stacking up, they gather strength, leaving you strung out and at risk of creating an exhausting, monster habit that becomes your norm rather than an occasional glitch.

'A habit is usually a sequence of behaviours, typically always occurring in the same order. It certainly requires very little conscious oversight,' Dr Kyle S. Smith tells me. An associate professor of psychological and brain sciences at Dartmouth College, Hanover, New Hampshire, he is an expert in the life of habits and how habits set up shop in our brain. 'Habits are done automatically,' he explains, 'and we might lump in obsessive or ruminative thoughts into that category that occur despite what you intend.'

Habits and thoughts

This confirms what Coué and Waters were on to at the beginning of the last century: that many habits are triggered by thoughts, because thoughts and the emotions we hug close set the stage for habits to put down roots; for example, that constant self-talk that tells you you're a terrible sleeper, you're going to wake up at 4am, that you're exhausted from lack of sleep, that you'll be awake half the night . . . these are all thought habits that are telling your brain what you expect to happen. But these suggestions, although powerful and often relentless, don't have to be given unlimited airtime; instead they can be challenged and shut down by consciously replacing any catastrophic or emotionally reasoned thoughts with others that are more balanced, factual and in tune with how well you *can* sleep with the right formula in place.

Habits exist to save us time, energy, head space and, in theory, to cut our stress levels, by rounding up a string of actions so that we can switch off from what we're doing to think about something else, whether you opt for that old favourite at the restaurant, buy yourself yet another dark blue shirt or take on a particular role when faced with a challenge, such as martyr, problem-solver or fly-off-the-handle person. Whatever situation we're in, the brain checks to see if it can pull a habit out of the hat to speed things up and make life that much easier for us. But habits can obviously work against us, if we don't stop to think: *Is this action actually doing me any favours? Do I really want to eat another chocolate while watching TV?*, or *Can I really survive on six hours of sleep a night? Does my brain have to see my bedroom as a temple to insomnia?*

Of course, the whole point of habits is that we *don't* stop to think. But sometimes we need to step back and give our habits a long, hard look. And if we don't like what we see, we can hack an old familiar habit that's become more of a hindrance than a help and switch it for a new one. They are that flexible.

Hot chocolate? Stale popcorn?

To discover how habits are hatched in our brain, and how one habit can be swapped for another, Dr Smith and Professor Ann Graybiel from the McGovern Institute for Brain Research at the Massachusetts Institute of Technology gathered rats, audio cues and tasty rewards. A T-shaped maze was set up to train mice and rats to take a left for chocolate milk or a right for sugar water in response to a sound cue. As predicted, the rodents got faster and faster as they learnt the drill, and the scientists found that the neurons in the part of the brain called the striatum fired up as the creatures got their heads around the challenge. But not for long. Once the rats and mice had got the hang of what was being asked of them, the scientists noticed that these same neurons only bothered to fire up at the beginning and end of the chocolate-milk or sugar-water dash to 'chunk' all the actions together, and they switched off during the middle, autopilot section of the action. The repetitions had left their mark: footprints in the rats' memories became deeper with every run. The instant the brain recognised the beginning of the behaviour pattern, it locked into an automatic neural response where the striatum could put its feet up and take a break. In other words: a habit was born.

Once a series of actions has been chunked together to create a habit in our brain, it also gets a coating of a fatty substance called myelin, which allows the brain's electrical signals to travel fast and smoothly, thereby making it an obvious, easy, go-to behaviour as well as harder to dismantle.

On a human level, we're all slaves to habit, without always realising it. Just the sight of a plate of food can cause us to pick up a fork and open our mouths obediently, without giving these actions a second thought. We rely on all manner of habits such as this to get us through the day. But while habits by their very nature go unnoticed under the radar (*Did I lock the door/turn off the stove?*), it's worth putting them under the spotlight occasionally, particularly when you realise that up to 40 per cent of our daily actions are carried out using our habitual autopilot. And habits, if left unchallenged, can be stubborn and hard to erase once imprinted in the brain's memory bank.

In *The Unbearable Automaticity of Being*, social psychologist, author and expert on the unconscious mind, John A. Bargh, and professor of psychology and neuroscience, Tanya L. Chartrand, argued that this running on autopilot is faster, effortless and inevitable, given the limitations of the conscious self, which is not able to maintain the effort required to keep a constant, vigilant eye on every move or decision we need to make.

A habit can turn into something we dislike

What's fascinating and very telling, when we think about the habits we've gathered over the years, is that even when the chocolate milk in Smith and Graybiel's rat experiment had been laced with something unpleasant tasting, the rats couldn't break out of the habit of running in that direction when given a certain audio cue. That's rats for you, you might think, but it turns out that humans will also cling on to a habit that's well past its sell-by date and not in the least bit tasty. Take the experiment carried out at the University of Southern California on a group of cinemagoers, who were chosen to take part because they *always* eat popcorn when they're at the cinema. Researchers found that as long as the members of this audience were allowed to eat with their dominant hand, they kept feeding themselves popcorn at the same pace, regardless of whether the popcorn on offer was freshly made and delicious or old and stale.

Rewards – chocolate milk, or fresh popcorn – give us a dopamine rush and make us feel good, euphoric even. This trains the brain about what is worth chasing and what is not. Does it want to go for a behaviour that comes with a lovely reward (in theory) or one that doesn't? There's no competition, obviously. But what if the reward becomes unappetising, or bad for us, but then we're stuck with the habit?

Fortunately, there's another part of the brain (the infra limbic cortex – IL cortex) that's keeping a beady eye on proceedings as habits take shape, and it's this part of the brain that decides if a habit is a keeper or not and which habit should be thrown into the ring in any given situation. Better still, if this part of the brain is turned off, we can come off autopilot, switch on cognitively (that is, make a conscious decision about what we want to do, rather than repeating the past) and freeze our bad habits, which can then be replaced. Old habits are effectively overwritten by new ones, and if we try out any new habit enough times, the IL cortex will grab at it, as it prefers a new habit to an old one, once it's learnt it and has got into the now-familiar routine.

Flashes of light into the brain (optogenetics) were used with the rats to temporarily turn off their IL cortex. The rats stopped in their tracks, came off autopilot, and were suddenly free to make a cognitive choice: did they *really* want to run in the direction of what had become an unpleasant reward, or did they want to start working on another habit by running in the opposite direction? Flashing lights into a human brain isn't an option (yet) for the general public, although a non-invasive technique that could be used on humans has been trialled on mice by a group of researchers in Tokyo, and research into optogenetics is ongoing. What is effective, research has found, is changing your routine and context cues, which will disrupt the beginning of the chain reaction and bring your autopilot to an abrupt halt. When it comes to sleep, that includes consciously challenging your self-talk, altering certain elements of your day to support your sleep drive, shaking up your sleep routine, transforming your sleep context/bedroom into a sleep haven and stripping your sleep countdown of stay-awake cues and loading it with ones that say 'Get ready to sleep tight.'

No favouritism here

Routine. Repetition. Cues. Reward – these are the four main building blocks that go into our habits, according to Dr Smith, which make habits simple to understand and very mouldable, especially once you realise that all habits are made equal as far as your brain is concerned.

With repetition, the more nights we spend wide awake, mind whirring with activity, or the more times we wake up ready to start the day at 4am, the more entrenched this sleep habit becomes. Repeat anything enough times and it becomes a habit.

Coué and Waters both clocked this need for repetition for a habit to stick, whether that was the Coué mantra of 'Every day, in every way ...' or other conscious auto-suggestions for specific problems. The Coué mantra was supposed to be rattled off 20 times, morning and night, in a 'monotonous and soothing voice', and the other auto-suggestions were also to be said again and again in the same way that a sleep script, listened to day after day, helps to re-write our sleep habits. 'The amount of impression which we can obtain by one direct suggestion is limited,' wrote Waters in *A Practice of Psychology*, 'while the amount we can build up by repetition is unlimited.'

With sleep that means consciously overlaying bad sleep auto-suggestions (plus routines and cues) with good ones and repeating this until they become our default setting and we've created a new groove for our neurons to fire along. Then we can lie back and watch as thoughts and/or words transfer into feelings, emotions, body chemicals and behaviour – and sound, energising sleep.

I managed to put an end to my 'bed is my time to think' habit by changing my routine and giving my thoughts an outlet with an armchair offload in a dimly lit living room just before bed. I also made sure that all my to-dos and work schedule were written down or in my diary so that I could tell myself (when in bed) 'That's all been dealt with, I don't need to go over that now. I can think about that tomorrow.' And I got my imagination on board to help alter my physiology and my reality, which we explored in 'What's willpower got to do with it?' on pages 28–30.

I also set up new cues – much like cognitive signposts – to help my sleep drive build up during the day. (This is our inbuilt need for sleep, which grows stronger as the day progresses if we don't disrupt it somehow, such as with long or ill-timed naps, chaotic schedules or too much artificial light, as previously mentioned.) My body and mind could then wind down for sleep at night. And if any stay-awake thoughts did sneak in and start making themselves at home after lights out, I'd switch them for a replacement habit, as discussed below, or use a technique called thought-stop (more on that later, in Chapter 5).

Forming a good replacement habit

During the day and pre-sleep, I tried to make sure that any self-talk reinforced the idea that I was going to bed *to sleep*. *Not* to lie around for hours with a wandering mind. I'd also remind myself of snippets from Waters' sleep script, which backed this up, and, together with the many sleep cues I'd set up, this mind-wandering habit was forced to take a back seat.

Not that this is *all* past tense. There is the odd night when I go to bed still *on* from the day, perhaps because I haven't given myself enough pauses or time to unwind, or my cortisol levels are too high, or my sleep pattern is messed up because I'm ill or worried about something, or I couldn't resist another episode. And then my old, after-dark thought habit tries to muscle its way back in. But this is no longer a real problem, at least not one that will keep me up half the night as before, because I can use the various tactics mentioned above, plus others I'll come to, to put the brakes on this sleep-wrecker of a habit, or to weaken it before it devours my night.

Distraction of the new

Do you get hyper-aroused? How about a tendency for negative or obsessive rumination, playing a negative thought track, sometimes on repeat? Do you get anxious/stressed a lot (leaving your body with too much cortisol)? And what sets that off? Do you have a fear of not being able to go to sleep? Or do you try too hard to sleep? Do you tell yourself that you're a hopeless insomniac? Do you saturate your nights with bright light? Do you work in bed (even if it's just in your mind)? Do you go from day to night to bed with no pause to wind down before you lie down? And the list goes on. Habits are sticky. And the brain loves the easiness of a habit, not bothering, obviously, to differentiate between a good habit and a bad one. Recognising what our bad sleep habits are, and being aware of what sets them off, has to be our starting block.

Hyper-arousal is very common in poor sleepers and insomniacs, because being hyper (as with too much caffeine) can stop you from easily winding down at night, thanks to all those action chemicals racing around your system.

The real breakthrough in the habit research carried out by Dr Smith and Professor Graybiel was the discovery that if you fracture the very beginning of a habit sequence, the chain reaction is broken, effectively creating a chink in our habit's armour and allowing any one of us to step in with a new desirable habit that supports who we want to be, or what we want to do. At this juncture it's worth emphasising that the brain responds to novelty, which snaps it into focus and off autopilot – so give it something new.

These days, if I do notice hyper-arousal, unwanted thoughts or stress-spike habits start to take over during the day (with all that cortisol that will ruin my sleep if left to accumulate), I break this habit chain by using various techniques; for example, I might change the cues and signals directed at my brain, re-read the situation I find myself in, swap my emotions, or take action that I know works to up my happy hormones and cut my stress. This will therefore stop more cortisol from being released and allow the stress chemicals that are there to subside – tactics that can make hyper-arousal unwind and evaporate, and stress spikes pop.

By removing cues that work against sleep, triggers for old routines are taken away, and old habits are left with nothing to set them off or for them to cling on to.

My daily routine that prepared me for sleep at night

With my new sleep routine, I stopped myself from lying around, thinking in bed in the morning, by throwing up my blind first thing to get the message across. I ate in a sleep-friendly way, with reasonably regular meals, to avoid sugar highs and lows, worked in tandem with the 24-hour clock, gave myself constructive suggestions and time cues, plus the daylight I needed, and I kept a close eye on my stress levels, ready to step in with appropriate stress-busters (as explained on pages 122–123). I also tried to adjust my reality, perceptions and emotions to suit. I listened to Waters' sleep script around 5pm, started dimming lights from 9–9.30pm to create a dusk zone, gave myself time to relax, or read just before going to bed (not always for that long), and I brushed my teeth by moonlight or by the dimmest setting on the dimmer switch. These were small tweaks and cues, among others that established a very new pattern where midweek I would go to bed around 10.30pm/11pm, be asleep 15–25 minutes later and wake up before my safety-net alarm, which went off at about 7am (although slightly later at the weekend). These days I can be more flexible with the time I go to bed, as I don't suffer from insomnia as I used to, although I do try to keep my hours as consistent as possible.

The huge thing for me, apart from not lying there for hours and hours at night, was that I woke up with energy, feeling strong physically and emotionally, rather than exhausted and worn out before breakfast.

Loading your nest with cues

It's the context cues – for example, those in your bedroom – that make *really strong* habits, so research shows, together with how many times the habit is repeated. With the rats mentioned earlier, sound cues were used to send them running left or right, but with humans, our multi-layered senses are simultaneously reading signals that are pouring in from all around, from sights, sounds, smells, touch, words, memories, thoughts and emotions, either pushing us towards a sleepless night or a deep, restorative sleep.

Sound cues work particularly well for some people. Music and sleep tracks (which, by association, can help you unwind before bed) prepare you for sleep and hold your hand as you move into sleep. Max Richter's full-length eight-hour *Sleep* is a soundtrack designed for people to sleep through what he calls his 'personal lullaby for a frenetic world'. Played live overnight, some of his audience listened to every note, others wandered about, while others snored away.

Once I appreciated how habits work in relation to sleep, and specifically how important the bedroom/context is, I set about fine-tuning my bedroom so that it was better prepped for sleep by removing bad cues and shipping in good ones. Anything to do with work was either put in another room, including a filing cabinet, or out of sight. I swept through, corner to corner, to minimalise as much as possible, adding a cover to the face of my bright digital alarm clock, a new comfy pillow and a soft pillowcase, a small, bargain barometer to keep an eye on the temperature and a pillow spray that diffused scents proven by neuroscience to aid sleep. All of this meant that my bedroom was now a relaxing, mess-free Ahhh space. Clear room, clear mind – with nothing around to engage it.

There are some cues that your brain really doesn't need to absorb: an uninviting bed; a 'wake-up' phone/tablet/screen/TV, tempting you to get online and engage mentally; a bright white bulb in your bathroom or bedside lamp; a desk piled with work inches from your pillow; any book/film/radio programme that makes you feel tense or over-engaged just before bed; a high-energy late-night snack; a light/noisy/hot bedroom; a late, animated or intense conversation that leaves you wired; a bright/tick-tock clock that makes you more aware of time than is helpful; and *I'm a rubbish sleeper who lies awake for hours each night* statements or thoughts. Any off-message, stay-awake cues like these need to be removed or avoided.

All in all, it was very gratifying to spring clean and streamline everything to be as conducive to sleep as possible, knowing that this was taking away props my old, negative, sleep habits relied on.

Helpful sleep cues

In contrast to work, clutter, bright lights and digital intrusion, sleep cues worth setting up as a magnet for new habits to stick to include:

- Evening loungewear, to signal it's time to unwind.
- A sleep-inducing soundtrack.

- A journal to empty you of pillow thoughts.
- Low, or red-spectrum lights for your bedroom and bathroom, as explored in the previous chapter (as we need light/dark cues to structure our day).
- A calm, quiet, dark, cool bedroom (I have black-out blinds and a dimmer switch in mine).
- A sumptuously comfortable bed that screams *me-time!* (reward).
- Clean bedding doused with Pavlovian sleep scents (this makes good use of the neuroscience of scent, which will be looked at in more detail in the next chapter).
- An artificial indoor dusk and night to consciously sync your body clocks and to let them know the countdown is on.
- Sleep-friendly thoughts and words.
- Deliberate biology-based suggestion/self-talk, supported by a sleep-script cue.
- A pre-sleep routine (however short and sweet).

Bedrooms need to be clear, tranquil spaces that are a relief to step into at the end of the day. A detox zone. Escape space. Private retreat. This is not a living room. It's a sleeping room – somewhere in which we can luxuriate that is not accessible to anyone and everyone, whenever *they* choose to make contact. Our beds need to be places for sleep, sex or sickness. And that's it.

A reward worth reaching for

'What really works in respect to habits beyond repetition is what we call reinforcement, so that would be something pleasant at the end – a reward,' says Dr Smith.

'The brain is really good and happy to form habits if it learns that something is going to be rewarding, so we're talking about having something very consistent that you do, with the same sequence, with a cue, and having a reward at the end – that's the strategy to form a new habit, or replace one that's problematic.'

Consistency and sequence. Cues. Reward. Repeat.

Creating consistency

Consistency in a sleep routine can come from any number of things; for example, creating a screen-free countdown and a dusk zone in sequence over the course of the evening, plus going to bed and waking up at roughly the same time each and every day, as much as possible.

Sleep cues can come from your routine, diet and environment, but also from a sleep script, out-loud auto-suggestions, well-chosen sleep triggers (sleepy scents and the like), or deliberate actions (deep breathing, meditation) or a biological body scan, once the lights are out. Then a reward can be thrown in to help it stick.

Rewards

We're all primed to be on the lookout for rewards or threats, whether that's us scanning for safety vs danger, a compliment vs criticism, a friend instead of a stranger or an arch enemy. Rewards help get us through the day. They're those little boosts or treats that keep us going, coming as they do with that dopamine hit – a euphoric, feel-good hit – which is why we want them so much, and why, conveniently, we can use them to cement our new-and-improved sleep habits, too.

Our brain prefers dos rather than don'ts (as Dr Syed Shariq Hasan explained to me). In other words, you're best off telling your brain 'Do this' instead of 'Don't do that', if you want results. This confirms Waters' positive approach to health: his belief that we should concentrate on our knowledge of the healthy body, and why and in what way it might be off course, rather than focusing too much on the illness. It's a constructive way of looking at things when it comes to rewards and sleep, too.

For example, we all know the risks we're running if we *don't* prioritise sleep, or if we *don't* give ourselves a decent screen break, or if we *don't* tune in to our body. But it's in our interest to focus on the upside, the health rewards, and what is going on in our body if we *do* give ourselves seven-plus hours of sleep a night, or if we *do* drink less alcohol and not right before bed, or if we *do* empty the brain chatter before lights-out, or if we *do* structure our day so that it leads inevitably to sleep.

We do, however, need at least to be aware of what our body's up against by not getting adequate sleep, so that we take our sleep life seriously. Too little sleep, for too long, increases the risk of heart disease, stroke, hypertension, weight gain, depression, obesity, diabetes, death and a weakened immune system, upping our risk of developing cancer, as well as reduced brain power, and accidents at work. Sleep deprivation also damages the eyes and doesn't give the brain enough time to flush out the toxic waste that has built up during the day – a toxic protein (beta amyloid) that's linked to Alzheimer's – which in turn pushes an exhausted brain into overdrive where it starts to eat itself. Not a pleasant thought.

If we can look at our healthy body and what is stopping it from getting the sleep it needs, however, we can reap all the rewards we gain from sleeping well or for long enough: a strong immune system, more energy, fewer health risks, maximum brain power, optimum equilibrium and well-being, less weight gain, balanced emotions and well-processed memories (the list goes on). This is obviously more appealing and less overwhelming than scaring ourselves with all the negatives that are on offer.

A day-to-day sleep reward is not necessarily something you can hold in your hand, although transforming your bedroom into a reward zone makes going to bed a reward in itself. It might be the fact that you feel calmer, stronger, rested, energised, healthier or just better about yourself, with improved sleep. For this you need to focus on how you feel come morning, so that the brain registers the reward that it's getting. You could give yourself a slap on the back for sleeping better than the night before – *I slept really well last night. I feel really good today. I slept much better than previous nights. I have loads of energy* – which makes for a very satisfying reward, in my experience. Or you could go for a more tangible reward by treating yourself to a delicious, sleep-friendly breakfast or morning snack.

Routine. Cues. Reward. Repeat.

Ditching and switching

A fifth habit-building block is the replacement habit. This is basically a stand-in habit. If you're trying to remove a habit, it makes sense that you'll need to fill the vacuum by replacing it with something else. The question you need to ask is, what would fill the gap for you? For smokers, nicotine gum can sometimes work. For compulsive snackers, clearing out the larder and switching high-calorie temptations for tasty, low-calorie alternatives is one option. For nail biters, gum, worry beads or fidget cubes can do it.

For sleepers, disruptive sleep habits need to be replaced with sleep-inducing ones. Do you lie awake for hours trying to *force* yourself to sleep? Or when you wake in the middle of the night, do you leap out of bed to watch TV, start working, listen to a gripping radio programme, surf the Net? Are you awake and clambering on the treadmill at 4.30am? Then stop. Look for habit stand-ins that can get you back to sleep: negative pillow thoughts can be replaced with that tried-and-tested well-being strategy of listing your gratitudes (which gets concrete sleep results after just a few weeks – increasing sleep duration by nearly an hour); and, rather than giving your brain a 'wake-up' activity and the message that it's fine to work at 2am when all is dark, relaxed meditation, mindful breathing, a quiet rest (in the dark) can fill what is a perfectly natural break between two sleep cycles.

Another replacement habit tactic you can use if your mind is determined to think about something in bed, is to run through what should be going on in your body as it gets ready to sleep, à la Waters, Dr

Sugarman and other practitioners of clinical hypnosis, to set off real cellular change. You can think: *My cortisol levels are down, and sleepy melatonin is up. GABA* (both a chemical messenger and an inhibitory neurotransmitter set off by darkness) *is shutting down my awake state* (for this I sometimes see dust-cloths being thrown over my synapses, to make them go to sleep); *my brainwaves are softening and slowing down and moving from beta to alpha* (which I visualise); *the deep breaths I'm taking are not only slowing my brainwaves, but they are also relaxing my nervous system and making my vagus nerve send the right messages to my brain that this is the time to rest and digest; my sleep-inducing neurons are piling up, ready to activate sleep's flip-flop switch.* Plus, just saying to yourself (in your mind): *I am going to sleep now*, is another surprisingly effective cue.

In your own time

I can't say how long, exactly, it took to switch my old sleep pattern for my new one, as I was experimenting with different factors as I came across them, rather than rebooting myself with them all at once in a more 360-degree fashion; however, all new habits take time to settle in, no matter if we hit the deck running or take it slow and steady, and regardless of how impatient we might be for change, with success coming in around day 18, 66, or 254 – to be precise.

These three numbers, far from being random, surfaced when 96 volunteers were put under the microscope as they very deliberately tried to forge new habits in a study on habit formation carried out on a group of European university students at the UK's Health Behaviour Research Centre. To find out how habits are formed, the volunteers were given the task of trying to set up new desirable habits by repeating a healthy eating, drinking or exercise behaviour, such as running for 15 minutes before dinner every day, or eating a piece of fruit with lunch, using situation cues as triggers, such as *before* breakfast or *with* lunch.

Over time and with all that constant repetition, the study found that the students' behaviour needed less and less thought, 'as control of the behaviour transfers to cues in the environment that activate an automatic response: a habit' (where the striatum could take a break). What also became clear over the months, as the 96 ploughed on, is that it can take a short time or a long time for a behaviour to become automatic and lodge itself as a habit – anything from 18 to 254 days, with the average being 66. This means that if disruptive sleep habits are still clinging on at night 19, there's no need to despair or give up. This is not a quick-fix, gaffer-tape solution. This is for the long haul.

Slipping up for a day, here or there, also has no long-term consequences and doesn't upset the efforts you're making to create a new habit, the study also discovered. That is to say, the odd sleepless night is nothing to panic about when you're ironing out your sleep behaviour – nor do you need to worry if you experience the odd crease further down the line.

Unfortunately, old habits never completely disappear. They're all in there somewhere; the new ones simply overlay the old ones, which, far from being eliminated, are simply loitering in the wings, weakened but on the look-out for a familiar trigger (cues, routines and contexts), which, if offered up, will act as an open door. 'We've done some neuroscience studies demonstrating this,' Dr Smith tells me, 'where you can take away a new habit and uncover the old one that was still there lurking. But the best way to prevent a resurgence is just being very aware of what the triggers are that caused it. Know what sets you off and know how to deal with it.'

If we can be wise to these old, lurking habits and recognise when an unwelcome habit is likely to grab at a passing cue, in order to resurface, then we can deliberately strengthen the new, replacement habit to make sure that this is the one the brain reaches for now and in the future.

I can see this sometimes when I go to bed too wired or preoccupied. My old sleep habits clearly jump with glee at the sight of a chance to take back control. But I'm aware of what's going on, and can counteract this, knowing that this is just a temporary blip with an obvious cause and one that I can sort out so that I can still get to sleep and wake rested. Routine. Cues. Reward. Stand-ins. Repeat.

---

4 top tips

1. Banish stay-awake habit cues from your bedroom, such as work and blue lights.
2. Load in sleep-inducing cues, such as sleep-triggering scents and red-spectrum lights.
3. Switch sleep-sabotaging thought habits for sleep-friendly ones.
4. Turn your bedroom into a detox haven: offline, phone-free and reward-heavy.

Chapter 5

How Do You Feel *Exactly*? Give it a Name. Any. Name. You. Like.

Stressful emotions rupture our sleep, unless
we can switch them for ones that suit.

Do you feel sad, cheerful, angry, frightened, bored, anxious or in love? Or do you just think you do? It's easy to overlook the fact that the names we give to different emotions are all made up. Different cultures give names and meanings to feelings and sensations that other cultures have never even heard of. But with every emotion releasing hormones into our body (some that help us sleep, and others that don't) being able to choose one emotion over another can really pay off.

'At any one time, there's a kind of flux of sensations and feelings [inside us],' says Dr Tim Lomas, senior lecturer in positive psychology at the University of East London and creator of the world's first positive lexicography compiled to help improve well-being. 'And we can stick a broad label on them, which they do approximate to, like anger or anxiety might feel broadly correct, but then actually we could be much more fine-grained and detailed about it,' he tells me. 'And the more people are able to be aware of their emotions and skilfully work with them, the better they'll be able to deal with things.'

This means we can either grab a generic emotion word that covers a huge range of feelings and sensations, such as anger, or we can zero in on the small print and benefit on many levels as a result. There is plenty of evidence to show that explicitly labelling and understanding our emotions doesn't just increase our well-being and reduce our stress but it can also improve our health and our resilience. This can clearly boost the quality of our sleep by reducing our stress hormones and giving our happy hormones a lift.

Take *tizita*, for example, the Ethiopian word for a bittersweet memory and a longing for a time, person or thing in the past, or *yilugnta*, Amharic for when we feel obliged to give in and agree with the opinion of others (even if we don't agree with them), or *wabi-sabi*, Japanese for the appreciation of imperfect beauty. There are many different emotion concepts to describe the subtleties of how we're feeling. If we can choose one that makes us feel less stressed or dissatisfied, for example, it stands to reason that our body chemicals and reality will change in line with that.

Anger, irritation, anxiety and depression tend to come with a shot of the stress hormone cortisol, which disrupts our chemical balance, our fluctuating melatonin levels and the ease with which we can get to sleep and stay asleep. As with replacement habits, which we discussed in the previous chapter, if we can look at the emotions we think we're experiencing and then swap them, if needed, for ones that work better for us, we can help to keep our stress levels down and turn around our days as well as our nights.

Saying, 'I feel angry' when we might on closer inspection be feeling frustrated, annoyed or insulted leaves us emotionally short-changed. It can also leave us facing the negative fallout that can come from calling out one feeling over another; for example, telling someone you're angry with them when you actually feel let down by their actions is likely to spark a very different reaction. If we can make use of more of the emotion concepts that are out there, especially the subtle ones that are loaded with nuance and encompass a variety of different feelings and sensations, experts say that we will be better equipped to deal with stress and bounce back more quickly from whatever challenges come our way.

Taking all this on board, I now question emotions that are winding me up or dragging me down, especially those that are spiking my cortisol levels, which I know will have a negative knock-on effect on my sleep if they are left to accumulate. And I try to look at my emotions in this unusual, more detached light, to stop stress chemicals from taking over and possibly ruining my day, and to embrace sleep-friendly emotions in a number of ways, which we'll now explore.

Murky is good

Ambiguous emotions are invaluable. These are those mixed emotions, where pleasant and unpleasant sensations are intertwined, and they've been underestimated for years in the West, sidelined in favour of the more black-and-white emotions that we often go for. Just as the emotion of hope combines a certain confidence that something in the future will happen with a bit of anxiety that it might not, the emotion of love can cover all kinds of feelings, some pleasant, and some far from it (fear, anxiety, vulnerability, for example), and the emotion of nostalgia can mix warm, fuzzy memories with a sprinkle of melancholy. Research shows that recognising the good as well as the bad in ambiguous emotions can help us to feel better about the bad bits and can raise our creativity as well as our resilience. And it's an emotional flip that anyone can do.

Adopting ambiguous or bittersweet emotions can effectively save us from ourselves. As one of my favourite new habits, this involves rejecting the idea that good/positive/happy emotions are the key to improved well-being, and that they sit at the opposite spectrum to bad/negative/sad emotions (rather than alongside them). And it scuppers the notion that we all have to try to force ourselves to be happy or more positive to achieve contentment, which is a pressure in itself. Instead, experts say, it's all about appreciating intermingled positive and negative emotions, and how expanding our knowledge of these ambiguous emotions is a healthy way forward.

Telling yourself that a cauldron of turbulent feelings is a mixed, or an ambiguous, emotion can make uncomfortable sensations pass much more quickly. I've found it stops them being blown out of proportion, or given enough attention to be interpreted as 'bad' emotions, with all the ramifications that can come with that. Plus, bittersweet, ambiguous emotions are right up there for reducing our stress levels, which in turn, of course, helps us to sleep better.

All well and good

Striving to be simply happy knocks out an appreciation of the more subtle, mixed emotions that can bring so much to the table. Instead, we're better off focusing on our well-being. Well-being is said to be rooted in:

- Having more pleasant than unpleasant moods and emotions.
- A general satisfaction with life.
- Autonomy (a feeling of control in your life, work, relationships, finances, etc.).
- Equilibrium.
- Meaning and a sense of purpose and fulfilment.
- Personal growth.
- Self-acceptance, based on an individual's aspirations (influenced by where you live and the people around you).
- Positive relationships with family, friends and all the other people in your life.

Work on these where you can, even in small ways and, needless to say, when well-being is up, stress, dissatisfaction and a lack of contentment go down. And you'll sleep more easily as a result.

The good. The bad. The ambiguous.

A detailed study called 'Bad is stronger than good', by a team of researchers based in Cleveland and Amsterdam, looks into how 'bad' always wins. It's eye-opening (and a bit of a wake-up call) to realise that bad comes out on top across the board, for a variety of reasons:

- Many more good deeds or events are needed to wipe out the memory of one bad one.
- Good reputations are hard won and easily lost, and bad reputations, vice versa.
- We get more upset about losing $50 than we are happy about gaining $50.
- We can ignore the beneficial things that people do to focus on what they don't do.
- One criticism is remembered over much praise.
- We have a lot more words for bad emotions than we do for good ones. Start counting and you'll see.

We can't help it. We're hardwired to focus on the bad rather than the good in life, which is believed to be an evolutionary leftover from the days when paying more attention to bad things could keep us alive. And this makes ambiguous emotions and a deliberate focus on good memories and positive emotions (however slight) that much more valuable, as well as making ourselves more adaptable and resilient, both for the small things and the big things; for example, at the end of a hard day, a relationship or even times of mourning.

By appreciating the 'good' side of mixed emotions, the 'Bad is stronger than good' researchers also found that we actually weaken the impression made by the 'bad' side. Go further and name your mixed emotions out loud and you can use spoken words to strengthen and solidify these thoughts.

In praise of the bittersweet

'Knowing more emotions can at least give people more tools for dealing with stress,' says Dr Lomas. 'It's fixed within the general area of emotional intelligence and emotional regulation, and the value to well-being of being able to appraise and manage your emotions, in terms of coping with them.'

Dr Lomas's positive lexicography (https://hifisamurai.github.io/lexicography), which is a collection of positive emotion concepts from around the world, allows you to browse emotions you might never have known you had – until now. And it gives a window on the world through the different emotions that different cultures live by.

There's *mono no aware* (Japanese), which embodies a beauty tinged with sadness: a sensitivity to and appreciation of the transience of things and the ephemerality of life and the beauty within that – the symbol of this being the short-lived first bloom of a cherry tree. Unambiguous emotions in the lexicography include *sisu* (Finnish), which refers to an extraordinary determination or courage, especially in the face of adversity; *mahalo* (Hawaiian) blends together feelings of thanks, gratitude, admiration, praise and respect; and *fernweh* (German), the 'call of faraway places' and the homesickness of the unknown. With so many of the world's emotions to choose from, suddenly the handful we tend to re-use again and again can look a bit thin.

Rather than rushing to claim a vague, 'umbrella' emotion, you can explore these emotion concepts, both from your own culture and others, in order to fine-tune how you read yourself. By deliberately identifying with emotions that are less broad (with many different meanings, to many people), black-and-white or gloomy, you can improve the quality of your life and save yourself from any unnecessary, negative repercussions that can come from choosing one emotion over another while keeping your internal chemical cocktail on a more even keel.

Emotion thoughts with concrete feet

By saying 'I am excited', as if you believe it, when you're in a state of high anxiety, before having to deliver on something (for example a piece of work, an exam, or a physical or social challenge), you are replacing any sense of threat with one of opportunity, argues associate professor Alison Wood Brooks, from the Harvard Business School, in her paper 'Get excited: Reappraising pre-performance anxiety as excitement'. You are, of course, also playing with your emotions to get a handle on those stress chemicals that can otherwise torment your sleep.

In Brooks's study, those taking part were given stress-inducing challenges: to make a persuasive public speech, or sing in front of a stranger, or tackle difficult maths problems – all of which were to be scored, with pulse rates monitored and with bonuses doled out for high achievement and extra pressure. Enough to spike anyone's anxiety.

Before each challenge, the participants were told to say, or in the case of the maths challenge, read, a statement that said that they were, or should feel: anxious, excited, calm, angry or sad. There was also a neutral test that gave them no prompt at all.

Now, motivational self-talk is nothing new. It's been used for years in business and sport, as an effective tactic to increase confidence and performance, and there are many scientific papers to back this up. Prior to Brooks's study, however, nothing had looked at how a self-statement about how you feel can actually *change* how you feel and transform your 'experience of emotion and subsequent behaviour'. No one had explored how deliberately misrepresenting emotions to yourself (that is, lying to yourself or changing the story) can effectively dupe your brain into believing that these emotions are the ones that you're actually feeling.

Say something out loud and you give extra weight to words that might otherwise have stayed floating around inside your head, so choose wisely. By vocalising your thoughts, you're not only bringing them out into the open, you're also creating your reality. Where a thought might fill your mind today, it can change tomorrow. But spoken words cement your thoughts, with consequences that you can't always undo – physically or socially.

In a pilot study of 300 people to find out what they thought was the best option for dealing with pre-performance anxiety, more than 90 per cent said trying to calm down was the best advice they could give. But they were wrong. Brooks's results were conclusive. Across the board, everyone who had the 'I am/get excited' prompt, performed over and above all the other participants. What's more, they actually *felt* more excited. This minimal intervention dramatically overturned the cognitive hit that comes with high anxiety. As Brooks's study wrapped up, 'The way we verbalise and think about our feelings helps to construct the way we actually feel.' Not only does this verbal trick use cortisol to the individual's advantage, Brooks believes that it could also create an I-am-excited, upward-spiralling success loop, while her experiment proves that a simple auto-suggestion can help disarm sleep's number-one enemy: anxiety.

'Our words codify and solidify our thoughts. Saying something out loud makes it more real than just thinking it in your head,' Brooks says, when I contact her to discuss her work, adding: 'Reappraising anxiety as excitement causes us to focus on the opportunities inherent in situations, rather than focusing on the threats. By focusing on opportunities and feeling excited, people smile more, feel energised instead of debilitated, and are more likely to succeed on both intrapersonal tasks – maths, writing – and interpersonal tasks: karaoke singing, public speaking, negotiating, seeking advice.'

*

Of course, it's obvious to those in the thick of it, that excessive anxiety torpedoes immediate performance (as well as your sleep). But what these experiments have shown is that just the suggestion of excitement can help you to up your game, and that re-appraising anxiety is much more effective than trying to crush it or urging yourself to feel calm.

Disarming a negative feeling with a positive one

I often use this now, whenever I notice that I'm feeling anxious about something. I tell myself that I'm excited by the challenge/situation/ future, rather than stressed or slightly terrified. 'This is really exciting,' rather than nerve-wracking or overwhelming, I reassure my brain, and then I feel my stressed-out cortisol levels re-cloak themselves in a much more useful, edgy excitement. And any worry, or feelings of dejection that might have come with the anxiety, subsides. Noticeably.

Disarm anxiety by turning it into excitement, and you also let your sleep quality rocket. Not only are you redirecting this cortisol to boost your immediate performance, confidence, focus and success, you're stopping your body from anxiously stock-piling it right up to bedtime, when it will aggressively stone-wall your attempts to relax and rest.

'Anxiety is a negative emotional experience,' Brooks tells me. 'There are physiological markers of anxiety – increased cortisol (stress hormone), heart rate, and skin conductance (sweaty palms). And there are psychological effects of anxiety – you spend time worrying and ruminating instead of focusing on the task at hand, which reduces one's ability to take others' perspectives; we rely too heavily on advice (even when it's obviously bad); and we are eager to leave conversations (even when staying in the conversation is obviously beneficial).'

Apart from switching emotions that have the same physical attributes, we can also reframe our emotions by looking at our feelings from a different perspective. 'We know that reframing distress as passion is helpful,' says Brooks, when I ask her what other feelings we can re-interpret to improve our day. 'For example, feeling upset at work is a reflection that you care deeply about your work. Following an expression of distress in the workplace (e.g. crying), research suggests that the way you label your emotions by saying, "I'm sorry, I'm just emotional about this" versus "I'm sorry, I'm just passionate about this" can profoundly influence how others view you. People who call themselves "passionate" instead of "emotional" are more likely to be hired.'

This is clearly where constructive self-talk and suggestion can come in.

If you're excited rather than anxious, you'll also be more optimistic about the possible outcome of challenges and more likely to take risks as a result, and your confidence and performance will step up. It's also worth examining your anxiety to see which sort you suffer from, as there's a difference between state anxiety, which most people experience throughout the day (when things gang up to stress you out) and trait anxiety, which comes down to personality and whether you're prone to getting anxious or stressed in certain situations.

Unfortunately, those of us who have trouble sleeping are liable to have trait anxiety *plus* state anxiety, the two feeding into each other, egging each other on. And insomniacs are said to be more susceptible to stress and 'tend to suffer from psycho-physiological hyper-arousal that prevents physical and mental relaxation', similar to chronic caffeine intoxication, according to a team of researchers from Switzerland, led by Dr Kyrill Schwegler. But armed with this self-awareness – the double whammy of two types of anxiety setting each other off – poor sleepers can take action.

I can now recognise when state anxiety starts to move in, often the result of stressors that come with juggling work and being a parent, when getting five minutes to yourself is something you often have to fight for. Is there some trait anxiety in there, too? Probably. But being able to rethink emotions, by re-reading feelings, sensations and the messages being sent to the brain, is an incredibly practical life tool that allows us to be more in control of our emotions rather than at their mercy.

Running with this idea of reframing of emotions, we can all help our sleep–wake cycle and the gathering force of our daily sleep drive by managing our stress levels via the words we choose to describe our many feelings. With a deep breath, I regularly:

- Swap anxiety for excitement.
- Dismiss unpleasant sensations as ambiguous, rather than worrying about the negative in there (nothing to see here).
- Recognise the good in the bad, to weaken the bad.
- Choose frustration over irritation at not being able to achieve as much as I want in a day, for example.
- Focus on appreciating what others bring to the table, instead of resenting what they don't.
- See low moods as the result of the need for social interaction or an early night, etc.

I know that if I change the signals coming in (a new location or a chat with a friend, for example), I'll change my feelings and my emotions. The aim of the game, for me, is to try to make sure that I won't be wired and loaded with cortisol or residual, unwanted emotions when I get ready to sleep.

Scrunch, scrunch

Performers and sports players don't only use suggestion and positive psychology to up their game, they also have all sorts of rituals they lock into before and during matches. It might be what they eat, or the order in which they eat it, before a game, or it might be how many times they bounce a ball before taking a free throw in basketball. The more elite the athlete, the more lengthy or elaborate the rituals tend to be.

And although most of us don't consciously reach for rituals to get us through the day, a simple ritual, it turns out, can be an extremely effective DIY strategy that asserts a sense of control over life and over any mounting anxiety. Pull out a ritual and you can bring your heart rate down and push your performance up; for example, in pre-performance situations, whether that's an interview, first date, exam, public-speaking event or sports challenge; or for dealing with the grief that comes with any loss, including the end of a relationship. I recommended this to my teenage daughter before an exam once, and she rated it enough to have used it since then.

To qualify as a ritual, our behaviour has to involve a repeated sequence of specific actions that are loaded with symbolic meaning. With placebo medicine, the ritual of meeting and talking with a doctor in a medical setting, the opening of a bottle of pills, swallowing a prescribed quantity at certain times of day, combined with all the rituals and symbols attached, all unconsciously feed into the hope and expectation that the drug will do its job, which sets in motion a positive placebo response. Prescription medicines, too, benefit from the placebo effect; for example, the placebo effect is thought to account for up to 45–50 per cent of the effectiveness of antidepressants, and was found to represent 50 per cent in a trial pitting migraine medication against a placebo (which all harks back to Coué's discoveries as a pharmacist). Also, the more faith a patient has in their doctor and the warmer a doctor's manner, the better the treatment will work. Even when patients know a medicine is a fake placebo (called an 'honest placebo'), the ritual involved and the expectation to get better that's wrapped up in that can achieve impressive results.

Whether your ritual is medical, or one that you've adopted or created, or one that's been given to you by a researcher, or even one that you are not actually aware of, they all work in the same way. You don't even need to believe in the power of rituals for them to benefit you, according to researchers led by associate professor Brooks.

In one experiment by Brooks's team, written up in 'Don't stop believing: Rituals improve performance by decreasing anxiety', the power of rituals to reduce anxiety was tested. Participants were told that they would be taught a new maths skill and then promptly tested on it: a high-stress, anxiety-inducing challenge. They were then split into three groups: one group was given a 'novel' ritual to carry out; one group was given a 'random behaviour' to perform; and one group was given no ritual or action at all.

And this is where it's interesting to see the power of words and suggestion come into play, as the ritual given to the first group was exactly the same as the random behaviour allocated to the second group, which was: 'Please count out loud slowly up to 10 from 0, then count back down to 0. You should say each number out loud and write each number on the piece of paper in front of you as you say it. You may use the entire paper. Sprinkle salt on your paper. Crinkle up your paper. Throw your paper in the trash.' But it was only those who were told they were in the ritual group who got better exam results. The symbolism and feeling of control wrapped up in the ritual wiped the floor with the 'random' actions, allowing this group to out-perform the others, as well as get a handle on their stress.

Feel it. And let it go

It's useful to be able to swap our emotions, as we've seen, but sometimes what's even better is to ignore them altogether. When it comes to emotional intelligence and knowing how to get the best out of our emotions, there are times when we're best off just sticking with the sensations going on in our body, rather than bothering to identify with any one emotion, which is where mind–body interventions such as mindfulness come in. If you can get into the moment with mindfulness, the idea is that you can reframe and let go of unwanted feelings, emotions and thoughts, especially those that are out of control or are dragging you down.

'Mindfulness is a time to be with the feeling itself, without all the mental elaboration – being sucked into unhelpful thought patterns and ruminations,' Dr Lomas, also an expert in mindfulness, tells me when we discuss emotions and mindfulness. 'It can bring you back to the present. I might have a feeling of anxiety and if I start ruminating on it, I'll get into all kinds of thought patterns. Whereas, if I was to just stay with the feeling, that might pass relatively quickly.'

Mindfulness – a 21st-century incarnation of meditation – is obviously one of *the* go-to de-stressers du jour. It's been gathering fans, momentum and medical kudos for years as an effective way to self-medicate for anxiety, depression and pain, and to offset the pace of modern life by anchoring everything in the moment and reducing all that noise for a few minutes or more. Whether that's walking mindfully, noticing the outside air or sun on your face, doing a mindful body-scan or eating a raisin mindfully (the classic mindful exercise), the aim is to get into the Now. And make everything go still – allowing the individual to have a different relationship with their thoughts and feelings. Less reactive. More observant. There are limitless things you can do mindfully to give yourself some down time. Mindful meditation involves closing your eyes and focusing on your breath. And if the mind wanders, as it's likely to do, you're supposed to just notice this and then bring your attention gently back to the breath, without reprimanding yourself for getting distracted.

It's big business, of course, with millions of app subscribers worldwide, but it's not *just* big business. Following your breath doesn't cost. What's more, just a few minutes can get results: calming both the central nervous system and the mind, and letting life's chaos pass you by at a safe distance. Are you sitting comfortably? Back straight, feet on the ground, hands on legs? Then all you have to do is close your eyes, feel your weight and follow your breath. In. And. Out. Even the briefest of pauses from life's rollercoaster can help you to catch your breath, unwind, secure some personal space, clear the mind of unwanted chatter and stop unhelpful thoughts, sensations and emotions from gathering momentum. Too simple? Research suggests that mind–body interventions (MBIs), such as mindfulness, t'ai chi and meditation, can do a lot for sleep quality, not least by soothing and even reversing the ramifications of stress at a molecular level by calming the bustle of genes that are wrapped up with inflammation (and inflammation, hyper-arousal and insomnia are all on the same team).

I don't do any lengthy mindful meditation during the day, just a few minutes of meditation at night, sometimes, to slow my brainwaves. But I do find mini mindful moments, or deep, mindful breathing for a couple of minutes, to be very effective for slowing everything right down, and stopping the mad dash of life (for a short while at least), giving my cortisol levels space to ease off and my mind some time to take a breath and unscramble.

Memories inhaled

Incredibly, 75 per cent of our emotions are triggered by what we smell. Scents not only release positive memories and feel-good endorphins, they can also improve our sleep, make us relax, lower blood pressure and heart rate, reduce pain, calm us down and alter our brain chemistry, moods and emotions.

The neuroscience of scent is set to take off, using, for example, placebo caffeine from piped coffee odours, memory kiosks to trigger feel-good emotions, and the digitisation of scents, where a digital smell could even feasibly be sent via the Internet (perhaps a holiday scent to go with that snap).

Studies show that peppermint, lemon and lavender all lower blood pressure and reduce the heart rate. Citrus scents can dramatically lift our mood and help to fight off depression. Rosemary boosts the brain to work faster and more accurately and also improves our mood. Lemon can make us feel thinner and lighter, vanilla can make us feel thicker and heavier, lavender has been proven time and again to help us relax, de-stress and sleep better, and chamomile, sweet orange, rose, ylang ylang and cedarwood can also all help us to unwind at night, ready for sleep.

Unlike with our other senses, the smells around us have a

powerful hotline to the brain. Neuroscience shows that the moment we inhale, those scent molecules are absorbed into our nostrils and at the back of our throat, setting off signals that are quickly sent to the brain, which responds by producing chemicals that go on to shape our emotions.

I sometimes use lemon essential oil while I work, and the zestiness of it seems to be a real brain pleaser. At other times I might go for rose (which makes me feel pampered, so it's a lovely reward), and occasionally I use lavender in the bedroom, to relax and sleep.

Olfactory experts well know that the impact smells have on our emotions and well-being should not be underestimated, although this is not something the majority of us are that focused on yet. But by understanding how different smells affect us physically and emotionally, we can either let our life and emotions be ruled by the smells wafting our way, or we can decide what smells we need when, and then boost our day with a scent menu that will alter our feelings, moods and emotions and take our everyday experiences to another level, as well as helping to keep our sleep stellar.

All alone in a crowded room

'There's loads and loads of evidence that the biggest killer is loneliness. However, you want to measure it – your happiness, your sense of well-being, your health, your ability to recover from diseases or from surgery, how long you live in the future, having got to whatever age you are now, is all massively affected by the number and quality of friendships you have, much more so than *anything* else, including underlying diseases. It is extraordinary,' says Professor Robin Dunbar, an expert in social bonding at the Department of Experimental Psychology, Magdalen College, University of Oxford, when I interview him for a feature about our need for eye-to-eye contact during the Covid lockdown and the virtual sleepovers that children were setting up to adjust to the challenging situation they found themselves in.

Loneliness is an emotional response that's often ruled by personal perceptions, but these can, fortunately, be turned around. For one, sleep loss and loneliness feed into each other in a vicious, mutually reinforcing loop. When we're tired, the brain is hypersensitive to potential social threats, perceived rejection or criticism and is less able to empathise with others, or read where they are coming from, which is why socialising can feel so uncomfortable and such hard work. Have you ever gone to a party or gathering exhausted? The chances are you couldn't relax, mingle or enjoy it as you would have liked, and you were left hovering on the fringe, misreading the social signals being given off all around you.

Being too tired causes an 'on-guard' attitude and with that comes negative social expectations that mean we're geared up not to click with or relax into social situations, before we've even entered a room. Instead, we give our brains the job of hunting out anything that might be construed as a rejection, social threat (hence cortisol spikes), or a negative social sign, to back up our lonely preconceptions. Catastrophic, negative thoughts can take over from rational ones based in fact. Rejected invitations become our 'failure' rather than the result of circumstance – for example, the person you approached/ invited was already busy that night; your text hasn't been immediately answered because that person is stressed, pre-occupied, on holiday, ill, working to a deadline, or having a digital detox, rather than ignoring you.

On top of this, sleep deprivation, or a lack of quality sleep, makes people more likely to avoid social situations in the first place, with this self-isolation feeding into their subjective feelings of loneliness and social isolation.

Studies show that other people look at sleep-deprived individuals and read them as lonely and therefore someone to be avoided, particularly as feelings of loneliness are contagious, making sufferers lonelier still. Loneliness also increases your stress chemicals at night, building another barrier between you and sleep that keeps you going round and round in a tired–lonely circle. Of course, if you are able to upgrade your sleep, little by little, you can weaken this sense of social isolation and loneliness.

There are four main interventions widely used today for reducing feelings of loneliness, and these are: increasing your social skills, social support, opportunities to socialise and changing your self-isolating perceptions. The most successful of these, it's been found, is changing our perception of the world around us: to look at life from the perspective of others and to empathise with what is going on with them, all of which works to calm our hyper-vigilance to social threat and help us to build resilience. A fifth intervention for dealing with feelings of loneliness is obviously the need to improve the quality of our sleep, to break the sleepless–loneliness cycle.

There's also an eight-week Mindfulness-Based Stress Reduction (MBSR) course that's been shown to relieve feelings of loneliness, not least by reducing the number of inflammatory genes, which tend to increase in lonely older people. Mindful meditation is believed to dilute the individual's perception of loneliness by reducing perceptions of distress or social threat, most likely by soothing the central nervous system, which is something you can also, of course, try out at home.

Also, by identifying distorted, negative thoughts, questioning them and then actively finding evidence that contradicts them, we can reduce any sense of threat and the sense of loneliness that comes with that. After all, loneliness can hit someone even when they are surrounded by the buzz of family and friends, or in the middle of a party, if they are not experiencing the connection they need. But we have to ask ourselves – what self-talk is taking place within? Are we ignoring positive social signs or memories to focus on misinterpreted 'negative' ones or unfounded future fears? Is that person really scowling at us, or are they just giving serious thought to what we've just said, or in a world of their own thinking about something else entirely?

Stop! That! Right! Now!

Medics don't advise that we ignore or suppress problems, anxieties, or intrusive thoughts that *have* to be dealt with, because they'll only come back to bite us later. Equally, though, allowing our mind to go over something again and again and again, in a circular, not-going-anywhere kind of way is not achieving anything either.

When it comes to sleep, thought-stopping can be a handy tool that can put a break on obsessive or intrusive thoughts that can set off negative feelings or sensations that then become our emotions. It's a gentle but firm way of holding up a hand to yourself to stop the chatter – a mental *shhhhh*. Worrying, obsessing, negatively fixating, playing a negative film reel in your head rather than a positive one, are not the same as problem-solving (which you don't want to do in bed, either), and there's nothing to be gained by locking into this mindset when lying in bed. Even stay-awake thoughts that are not negative, such as planning tomorrow or next week's to-do list, or your next holiday, need to be stopped.

I've found that it can be very effective to just say: *Stop!* (in my mind), *Enough of that. It's time to sleep.* As I have already said, ruminating used to be one of my worst sleep habits, and it is the same for many people. If we don't pause or catch our breath during the day or have any alone time, going to bed can become that time of day when we give ourselves a window to reflect, ruminate and solve problems.

The cue 'Stop!' is effective because it distracts you (breaking that habit sequence) and because it is recognised by the brain as a ticking-off and a 'punishment-orientated command'. By punishing yourself when you find unhelpful thought patterns or sleep-blocking thought loops taking over, you weaken the habit. The more frequently you do this, the more effective the cue.

Thought-stopping has also been used for years in the sports world as a cue to stop any negative, undermining thoughts from taking hold. And it's said to be even more effective when followed by something positive or reassuring (which is where repeating your gratitude list can come in, or focusing on the rewards of a good night's sleep – to fill the habit vacuum that's appeared). Or you can use mental techniques, such as recognising and rationalising what are called unhelpful thinking styles, such as:

- All-or-nothing thinking (where everything is seen as one extreme, or another).
- Magnification or minimisation (where we magnify the positive attributes of others while minimising our own).
- Catastrophising (blowing things out of proportion).
- Emotional reasoning (where we think that what we feel is true).

Attempting to recognise and rationalise these thinking styles is a tactic that you might want to try out during the day so that you're more equipped to disengage mentally at night.

Mind-wandering is also bad for us. In an interesting study, 2,250 adults had their thoughts, feelings and actions tracked using an app to jump into their day at random moments (known as experience sampling). The app asked them what they were doing right then, and if they were thinking about that or something else, whether pleasant, neutral or unpleasant, and how good or bad they felt. What researchers found is that humans love to let their minds wander, which happened 46.9 per cent of the time the 2,250 people were contacted, with their minds wandering towards something pleasant 42.5 per cent of the time, towards something unpleasant 26.5 per cent of the time and neutral 31 per cent. What's more, thinking about something pleasant did not make them feel happier than if they had just focused on whatever they were doing in the moment, whereas neutral and unpleasant thoughts made them feel much unhappier. The study concluded that mind-wandering causes unhappiness rather than unhappiness causing mind-wandering.

So with roughly 50 per cent of us daydreaming at any given moment – and nearly 60 per cent of those mind-wanderings making us feel worse, and the other *c.*40 per cent of mind-wanderings, although pleasant, making us feel no better than if we were just concentrating on the moment – what has been shown is that mulling over the past, present or possible future (rather than the moment), or spacing out into fantasyland, doesn't come with a feel-good factor or any benefits to our well-being. We'd be better off using thought-stopping and focusing on the here and now, and when it comes to bedtime being strict with ourselves, banishing wandering thoughts, with all the feelings and emotions that they can cause, by using the punishment-orientated command, 'Stop. Now is not the time for all that. Now it's time for sleep.'

I'll have that one, thank you

There are trillions of cells in the human body, and those in the nervous system are constantly firing off in response to what's happening to us, urgently whispering to each other at lightning speed to communicate how we're being affected by our immediate environment. The brain reads the signals, looks at the emotions on offer and makes a judgement call. But given that anger and fear are physiologically the same, as are excitement and anxiety, ambiguous emotions are often overlooked. Because we can only classify our emotions by using the concepts stored in our brain's dictionary of emotions, it's easy to see how we might opt for one emotion over another, at our expense, especially if we're tired or have not given ourselves enough time to pause.

In *How Emotions Are Made*, Lisa Feldman Barrett argues that emotions are far from hardwired. There are no specific areas of the brain that are dedicated to different emotions, and although we might all use the same emotion words, such as angry, happy or depressed, we don't always use them to mean the same thing. According to Barrett's theory of the constructed emotion, our emotions are our brain's best guess for what all that sensory input means at any given moment, and it uses our past, the concepts we know, physical sensations going on and what's happening around us, before making a choice. As she puts it, 'You are not a passive receiver of sensory input but an active constructor of your emotions. We are architects of our own experience.'

I saw this in action one time when my brain read my aching limbs and a general chill as an on-coming cold, until I wrapped up and remembered the workout I'd done the day before, which made my apparent cold symptoms suddenly disappear. Likewise, where I might before have felt a bit flat or overwhelmed by life and its never-ending to-do list, which might later keep me awake, I can now choose to change the sensory data I'm working with: by swapping the four walls around me for whatever's going on outside, packed with different images and stimuli.

Are you feeling glum and lacklustre? Slumped and inactive? Sore eyes? With nothing going on? Your brain can read the signals. It puts two and two together, and ... you must be a bit depressed, filled with self-doubt or under the weather; it's time to lie down with a dejected attitude and a cup of cocoa. Alternatively, whether glum, slumped or not, you can take the decision to re-read the signals, feelings and emotions, or get proactive and throw some different cues into the mix to spoon-feed your brain an alternative message, which works because the brain responds to novelty. This is all about offering yourself the best, most advantageous emotion concept that you can think of (or learn) for whatever sensations you're feeling or the situation you're in.

This might be a very different way of looking at emotions for many of us, but if we can alter our emotions for the better by choosing our emotion words carefully and re-reading our physical sensations or the emotions that we think we're experiencing, then this is clearly a useful life skill to have. And if we can consciously re-focus on different cues, memories, perspectives (including other people's) or move our body (sit straight, stand proud, dance on the spot, stretch, change location, go for a walk, climb out of that rut, surround ourself with new smells, sights and sounds), this can help us make the shift. In this way we can shake things up and change the cues and the messages that are bombarding our brain and the predictions it will make as a result, as well as adjusting our perceived emotions, reality, stress levels, body chemicals *and*, therefore, the quality of our sleep.

4 top tips

1. Re-read feelings, sensations and emotions to your advantage.
2. Recognise the good, as well as the bad, in mixed emotions.
3. Learn some new emotion concepts that speak to you.
4. Change the emotion-generating messages being sent to your brain.

Chapter 6

Slow Down, You're
Moving Too Fast

Our sleep doesn't stand a fighting chance without
science-based stress-busters to throw into the ring.

Stress can be useful, in small doses. If you channel it right, it can sharpen the mind and get the adrenaline pumping so that you strive to achieve your best. But when work deadlines, money troubles, chores and family commitments keep coming at you, and then digital communication overload begins raining down. That's when it can get out of control. Your stress chemicals can shoot up to dizzying heights, and your day-to-day acute stressors tip over into chronic stress, which can, in turn, lead to debilitating anxiety and depression.

The fact is that we all need to step back from the speed and stressors of modern life and make time, however brief, to slow things down a bit. To pause. Unwind. Reconfigure. De-stress. And to bring our cortisol levels down, and, as result, improve our health, equilibrium, the chemical cocktail within us and our sleep.

Figh or flight, as we know, is supposed to be a short, sharp adrenaline-fuelled reaction that takes over when we're faced with a threat, a challenge or a stressful situation. But it's also supposed to melt away when that danger is averted or the challenge dealt with, giving our bodies and minds time to recover, kick back and de-stress. And while anxiety is our internal, emotional reaction to stress, stress is triggered by *external* causes: what's going on around us. The problem with external stressors is that they don't always stop.

Even without stressors, let alone any real physical danger, our imagination can set us off. We can get stressed about being stressed: fearful of fear, eaten up by future worries, sick or anxious at the thought of another sleepless night. Trapped in this mindset, and the emotions we've honed in on, we can have a job of trying to settle into rest and digest, and subsequently wind down into a deep, tranquil sleep as quickly as possible and to stay asleep.

As Waters put it:

> Let us suppose now that fear is active in the mind and therefore is over-stimulating these glands, but that the physical efforts are not needed because the fear is an abstract one called into being by memory, or fear of some event distant in time or space. The extra sugar is now not needed and not consumed ... The physiological becomes pathological.

Meaning that out of sight, below the surface of our skin, rest and digest is effectively being outgunned by fight or flight, and sleep kept at bay or disrupted by adrenaline and all its stressy, chemical pals.

Even mild stress, if it's relentless, can push our cortisol levels up too high, making us wired and hyper-aroused – cognitively and physiologically – preventing us from switching off easily when we go to bed, from sleeping soundly, or forcing us awake too early in the morning. And it's hardly a coincidence that insomniacs have excessive amounts of cortisol charging about their bodies at night. That's a concentration of our action/stress hormones at a time when we need our brainwaves to slow down and a go-to-sleep missive to start purring its way around our system. But instead of saying, 'It's night-time. Get ready to deactivate. Slow down and prepare for sleep', the message is clearly saying, 'Stay alert and hyper-vigilant. Just in case.' And our HPA stress-response trio can't help but respond to that.

Stress-busters

To deal with this, I've gathered a wide range of science-based, stress-busting, mood-boosting tactics that we can turn to, to counteract the stress in our life, many of which involve the extraordinary power of suggestion. For one, it's worth remembering that humour and laughter release feel-good hormones, reduce stress hormones and anxiety, strengthen our relationships (by bonding and defusing tension) and are very effective coping mechanisms (even, it has been found, for firefighters who are managing a traumatic job). Reading a paper book cuts stress by up to 68 per cent; looking for the good in the bad (such as the creativity, connectivity and acts of kindness that came out of the Covid-19 crisis) helps to boost your resilience; giving yourself a pause during the day, just to switch off, allows your stress chemicals time to subside; and learning to embrace ambiguous emotions, or re-write your emotions altogether, can alter your reality in seconds. All of the above can be used as and when they're needed or to take pre-emptive action to stop the stress chemicals from escalating and then tipping the balance.

There's no question that I used to be more stressed than I am now, but again, as with sleep, I had no objective perspective I could take before researching for this book, no tools to disarm it and no biological insight. I just lived with the fallout, which could upset my day, and, of course, without me knowing it, disrupt my sleep.

Stress has been declared a 21st-century health epidemic, with the financial crash, climate change and social media given as three of the main causes (before Covid came along). In the UK, nearly 50 per cent of our sleep problems are directly blamed on stress, according to the Sleep Council's Great British Bedtime Reports, while 74 per cent of Brits said that their stress levels were so high that they felt overwhelmed or unable to cope in a 2018 poll carried out by the Mental Health Foundation. A survey by MIND found that one in three people (34 per cent) are stressed by work, 30 per cent by debt or money worries and 17 per cent by health concerns, with over-the-counter sleep aids and prescription sleeping pills used to help cope with this. Americans rank among the most stressed people globally, with nearly 77 per cent struggling to sleep during the coronavirus outbreak.

If we can tackle our acute, in-the-moment stress, however, as well as any ongoing chronic stress that can snowball into anxiety, using even the smallest of coping mechanisms to relieve some of the pressure, we can help redress the body chemicals that are messing with our health and our sleep. We can then stop ourselves being sucked into this adrenaline-cortisol-filled whirlpool. Because the reality is that we simply can't run around all day being highly stressed, anxious or overstimulated. Stop. Lie down. And then expect quality sleep to quickly follow and stay with us for the whole night.

A stress present, wrapped with a bow

Some people are lucky enough to be genetically predisposed to being less stressed, thanks to the effectiveness of a chemical called neuropeptide Y (NPY), it's thought, which is seen as a sort of on–off switch for the individual's stress-response system. Even without this inbuilt advantage, research shows that if we can change how we *perceive* stress (seeing it as enhancing, rather than debilitating), this will affect how we actually *experience* stress.

The Stanford Mind and Body Lab at Stanford University, California, put together a series of three-minute videos that were biased to present stress as either debilitating or enhancing. The researchers proved that it is possible to change the way stress affects us in just 180 seconds (https://mbl.stanford.edu/instruments/

stress-mindset-manipulation-videos). The 'debilitating' video states, 'Your focus is at its worst under pressure.' With an image of someone with their head in their hands, it says 'even the smallest amount of stress can hinder cognitive performance', adding that our body's stress response can deteriorate our focus, decision making, memory and performance, and ending with, 'Stress is deteriorating. Learn to manage it. Learn to avoid it.'

In contrast the 'enhancing' video opens with footage of a runner, overlaid with the message 'Most people assume that in order to perform at the highest level, you need to be calm and stress free. But, in reality, it is pressure that fuels peak performance.' And it goes on to give examples of how brain function can be heightened by stress. Ending with, 'Stress is enhancing. Utilise it. Let it improve your performance.'

With the team's stress-is-debilitating video, there was no change in the viewers' outlook, because that's the message that's all around us and the one the majority of us live by. But with the stress-is-enhancing video, researchers found that they could actually transform the way we look at challenges by making us see stress as an indispensable tool that can get us from A to Z. What's more, they discovered, those with a stress-is-enhancing attitude had only a moderate cortisol response to stress, as opposed to a high one, and a more positive attitude in general.

For those unable to feel the enhancing potential of their stress, there's a very logical and effective strategy to change your relationship with stress, devised by clinical psychologist Dr Alia Crum, who is head of the Stanford Mind and Body Lab. I have paraphrased her three steps for rethinking stress – by acknowledging, welcoming and utilising stress – mentioned in her lecture at the Gladstone Institutes (https://www.youtube.com/watch?v=4z9clzqhCN0). It goes something like this:

1. First, we need to acknowledge our stress (I'm stressed about –, because –). The science behind this being that by acknowledging *what* exactly is stressing us out, we

move these stress-wrought thoughts that can become all-consuming and debilitating, without ever moving forward, from the highly emotional and reactive amygdala region of the brain, to the more cognitive and reasoned pre-frontal cortex. And once we've shifted these thoughts to the pre-frontal cortex, we can think more clearly about what is stressing us out and what we can do about this.

2. With our stress relocated to the pre-frontal cortex and, as a result, more under control, the next step is to embrace the stress (rather than trying to dodge, ignore or suffer it), recognising that the only reason we're stressed out in the first place is because it's about something we really care about. We might be stressed about reaching a particular goal, getting the results we need, or because there seem to be too many obstacles in our way, or simply about being late for an appointment, or something we want to do.

3. And, lastly, we need to utilise our stress to secure the reward we're after, whether that's meeting a deadline, passing an exam, getting some headspace, or a promotion, being a great parent, earning enough to pay the bills/improve our quality of life, or striking something off the daily to-do list … as that shot of adrenaline will help drive us forward.

Reminders for this could be: stress makes me faster and more focused. I am only stressed because I care about what I'm trying to do/achieve. Stress is an enhancing tool that I can use to my advantage. Stress is helping me to meet these challenges (such as being asked to do too much in too short a time). These positive suggestions (aka self-talk/self-hypnosis), repeated for maximum effect and to change habitual thoughts, work to cut our stress and our cortisol levels, by profoundly altering our perception of stress.

A cup of happy hormones, anyone?

Are you fed up? Burnt out? Disgruntled? Stressed? Depressed? And carrying all of that to bed with you? To change the story and cancel out daily stress we can activate the four happy neurotransmitters, those smiley-faced chemical messengers that we all want plenty of: dopamine, serotonin, endorphin and oxytocin. If we can get those up and running, they'll feed into each other, helping to keep us healthy and content, and in turn optimising our sleep.

The fact that depression can lead to insomnia and insomnia can lead to depression, with 97 per cent of those who are depressed reporting sleep difficulties, and depression declared to be 'the leading cause of disability worldwide' by WHO, deliberately boosting our happy hormones can help to counteract this negative loop on a very practical level.

1 **Dopamine** is that euphoric rush we get with a reward or something we like, be that a hobby, compliment, delicious food, glass of wine, good company, mindful moment, crisp, clean sheets, and the like. It's why a reward at the end of a habit chain makes the habit stick, training the brain to chase the reward. It's also why regular mini rewards throughout an overwhelming task or day will keep us pressing on. By looking for the possible rewards in any situation, however challenging, you defuse any sense of threat and put your brain into approach mode, with a more I-can-do-this attitude.

2 **Serotonin**, the antidepressant, comes from the following: putting yourself in a good mood, feeling significant, dwelling on your achievements and self-worth, having positive social interaction, receiving bright vitamin-D-saturated daylight (or mood-enhancing blue-white lights, or the light given off by a light box if daylight is in short supply), the smell of essential oils such as lavender, bergamot and lemon, and a tryptophan-rich diet (see pages 145–146). All of this helps with sleep, because 'happy' serotonin is needed for the production of 'sleepy' melatonin.

3 **Endorphin**, a morphine-like anaesthetic, is the brain's answer to physical pain and stress, that dulls anxiety and the perception of pain, and is released with exercise, as well as laughter, singing, chocolate and spicy foods.

4 **Oxytocin** is best known as the 'love hormone'. It is linked to improved sleep, well-being and mental and physical health, but it specifically has an inhibitory effect on stress: it calms and repairs the body, is believed to help with feelings of trust and our ability to read other people, it stimulates growth and healing, and is released in response to sensory stimulation (skin-to-skin contact, hugs, stroking an animal, social interaction, rest and relaxation, massage, sex, holding hands, childbirth, breastfeeding, warmth, food, conversations that count, altruistic acts, a warm bath) in a safe and reassuring environment.

Being aware of these four happy hormones has made me much more conscious of what I can do to keep my body chemicals in a good place, and more reward-focused. Being outdoors is a big one for me, surrounded by trees and green open spaces: early morning walks, Sunday hikes or day trips and rowing on a river when outside of the city (although you can do this too in many urban parks). Also great are family chats in front of a roaring fire, an evening with a friend, a new book, a glass of something delicious, a wander round an art gallery, a funny movie (which can change emotions, de-stress and boost the immune system), with a calm, comfortable and (ideally) clutter-free bedroom as my reward at the end of the day.

You might opt for a mindful pause, a lunchtime stroll, time alone listening to music or playing an instrument, doodling, painting, birdwatching, doing some gardening, going for a coffee, having a foot spa, or whatever reward or happy hormone triggers work best for you. They will all reduce your stress chemicals, making it easier for you to sleep well at night. Studies also suggest that helping or caring for other people, rather than ourselves – for example, by volunteering or carrying out random acts of kindness – can be even more successful for boosting our feel-good moods.

Thank you. Thank you

Listing some of the things you're grateful for in life might sound like a wishy-washy card to play but it gets proven results when it comes to enhancing sleep and strong-arming unhelpful, brain-monopolising thoughts out of the bedroom door (so that you can deal with all that – if you have to – in the morning). By thinking about everything you're grateful for, you are switching your focus away from any stress-inducing thoughts towards rewards and giving your serotonin levels a boost. By substituting a gratitude list for gripes, you also free yourself from negative ruminations that can stir up all sorts of unhelpful physical sensations and the body chemicals that come with them.

In a study titled 'Counting blessings versus burdens' carried out by the University of California, Davis, researchers found that people who took the time to list the things in their day that they were grateful for every day for three weeks (even little things counted) not only improved their mood and energy but also the quality of their sleep and the amount of time they slept – by an impressive 52 minutes a night.

If you can give yourself time to think through or write down anything that you're grateful for some time before bed, this minor intervention can effectively influence the way you feel, increasing positivity and reducing negativity. Even your partner will apparently notice the difference this makes to your sense of well-being and satisfaction with life. What's more, the University of California's study discovered that this works for everyone, regardless of age, sex, personality or what is going on in their lives.

I used to do this much more regularly as part of my sleep countdown when I was sorting out my chronic insomnia: after listening to a sleep script early in the evening, during my pre-bed armchair offload, or before/after reading a book. But I still find it very effective sometimes when I'm in bed to help me unwind or to stop my mind from thinking/fixating/worrying about things when it should be switching off.

If you're inclined to lock into habitual, negative thought loops (or even positive ones), particularly when you're lying in bed, you can nip this habit in the bud by pulling yourself up short when you find you're doing this, and then fill the habit vacuum by thinking instead about the things you are grateful for, which will disrupt and re-route this bedtime habit, sending it off in the direction you want it to go.

Do I look bothered?

Other people can sometimes be a problem – or our reaction to them. People can stress-dump, for example. But that doesn't mean we have to absorb what they're dumping. If they're not stress-dumping, they might just be winding you up, rushing you unreasonably (or you might be rushing yourself), leaving you with hurry sickness (from the German term *Eilkrankheit*) or doing a time-grab – of *your* time. Whichever it is, you need to buffer yourself, ring-fence your space, time and equilibrium, if you can, and stop your stress chemicals from being triggered.

Émile Coué had a 'Do I look bothered?' kind of approach. He urged nipping any rising annoyance in the bud, by saying to yourself, 'No, that does not trouble me at all.' It's a tactic that's surprisingly effective, I've found, as my brain seems to respond with a slightly startled, but relieved, 'OK. I'll switch off from that then.'

Page by page

Curling up with a good book in a quiet corner is effective for reducing stress on several fronts. Losing yourself in a book not only cuts stress, it also relieves depression, upgrades sleep and sharpens the brain by stimulating it on many levels – not least the fact that you need to remember the plot and characters every time you pick it up – and it provides some peace and quiet, giving you a break from noise pollution (which is becoming a real health hazard).

Reading a book also increases our well-being and ability to empathise with others. A six-minute read is enough to slow the heart rate, relax muscle tension and cut stress by 60 per cent – like going on a mini break from wherever you're sitting. And if we read a book for 30 minutes or more in a day, it can help us to live longer – 20 per cent longer than those who don't read books. The longer you read, the better the benefits. Reading is also an effective sleep-habit cue and a perfect stepping stone between day and night, helping us to unwind from, and draw a line between, a hectic day and our countdown to sleep.

Stress and its chemicals can be intercepted and manipulated so easily with a quick read, so that they don't take hold of your day and night. This is just as well given that, apart from disrupting sleep and our all-important body clocks, too much cortisol not only suppresses the immune system but also leads to high blood pressure and excessive, adrenaline-driven sugar levels, which can cause diabetes, weight gain and mood swings. Plus ongoing stress, with its fearful chemical responses, leaves the body and neurons worn out and at risk of all sorts of other illnesses.

Noise, in contrast to books, raises our cortisol levels, increasing our blood pressure, and has been linked to a number of illnesses including cardiovascular disease, type-2 diabetes and depression. Not only can it stop us from getting to sleep, but it interrupts our sleep because we can still hear when we're in a light NREM sleep. The European Environment Agency has found that there are more than 10,000 premature deaths and 900,000 cases of hypertension a year, in Europe alone, due to noise pollution, with millions suffering from sleep disruption and nearly 6.5 million suffering high sleep disturbance thanks to the cacophony going on around us (the most constant offender being road traffic). Silence, however we can get it, is something to treasure, or create.

Even stressed-out whales were said to benefit from the drop in noise pollution from passing ships during the spring 2020 coronavirus lockdown. I often wear earplugs while working, to cut out distracting urban (or household) noises that can break my concentration and trigger stress, and I generally keep things quiet just before bed, with low-volume background music, TV, or silence and a book. Noise-cancelling headphones are another option people sometimes go for during the day, as are white-noise machines at night, plus insulation and quiet spots away from the crowds, when possible, are worth prioritising to give your ears a break.

Move your body

The other big stress buster is, of course, exercise – a real stress-relief valve. With endorphins guaranteed. And even a short daily burst gets worthwhile results. I go for early morning walks as often as possible, getting my dose of morning daylight at the same time, and I stretch and strengthen with at-home Pilates and a tick-list to work through all the muscle groups. I could do a lot more, obviously, but I'm working on that.

The latest is that we should just keep moving instead of stagnating. Five minutes here and there, scattered throughout the day, and using no more than our body weight, and possibly a step, wall or raised surface, is enough to get our muscles firing. Our bodies need regular movement, and little and often works well. We create our own energy, after all. But it's the moderate-to-high levels of exercise that are truly effective when it comes to redressing poor sleep, studies have shown – as long as you don't exercise just before bed, which will leave you energised and hot when you need to wind down and be cool.

Exercise helps us sleep, thanks to the drop in stress and anxiety levels that comes with physical activity, plus the increase in endorphins as well as serotonin, which our bodies need to produce the sleepy hormone melatonin, and then there's the antidepressant and anti-inflammatory effects of a good workout, too.

It can be hard to keep up an exercise regime, but you could always set up a few habit cues as prompts or to keep you on track; for example, you could lay out your gym kit somewhere it can't be missed, or where it will be ready to be put on first thing; you could link exercise to times of the day – for example, do five-minutes of stretches before getting dressed in the morning, a few wall press-ups, squats or lunges before every meal, or arrange early morning walks with friends. Other habit cues are regular workouts, team sports (which are said to strengthen the five C's: competence, confidence, character, connections and compassion/caring), or classes with others so that you are tied into a commitment (dance-fitness classes, such as Zumba, are a fun option); try to take your gym kit to work and head home via the gym, or just jog back – and keep repeating these exercise cues and routines, however minimal, with suitable rewards, until they become a habit.

Exterminated by the plant

Walking is widely undervalued, despite being an effective mood-lifter, with scientific backup. No gym membership is required, and it's not only one of the easiest forms of exercise to fit into our day but it cuts stress and boosts our immune system, too.

Active commuting – using your legs rather than wheels to get to work – or a morning speed walk to soak in that early daylight, a quick lunch-time blast round the block with a pedometer to gee you on, or any other opportunity you get to walk. Anything is a bonus, particularly as walking has been found to have no damaging effects on the body. It improves cardiovascular health, burns energy at any pace, increases bone and muscle strength, lowers stress hormone levels and blood pressure, upgrades sleep and aerobic fitness (as long as your breathing rate speeds up, you turn red and sweat a bit), and that's not to mention the positive effects it has on your everyday well-being. And the faster you walk, the better the physical results.

*

Forest Bathing, or *shinrin-yoku*, was first launched with Japanese government backing in 1982. Taking in the forest atmosphere is growing in popularity and has been scientifically proven to significantly diminish stress and depression, strengthen the immune system and increase energy levels. And the more stressed you are, the greater the payback.

Essential oils released by the trees and plants, called phytoncides, float around in the forest atmosphere, and when you inhale them you hike up your body's store of natural killer (NK) cells that attack and destroy virus cells. The phytoncides are also linked to a strong immune system and the body's defence system against cancer, according to research carried out at the Nippon Medical School, Tokyo. Phytoncide, which means 'exterminated by the plant' and is otherwise known as the aroma of the forest, is given off by trees and plants to protect themselves from germs and harmful insects. Fill your lungs with this potent air on a trip to the woods and you significantly increase your NK cells for the whole of the next week, while the positive effects of the trip will last for a month.

A vast field experiment into the physiological effects of *shinrin-yoku*, carried out across 24 Japanese forests, found 'forest environments promote lower concentrations of cortisol, lower pulse rate, lower blood pressure, greater parasympathetic [calm] nerve activity, and lower sympathetic [not calm] nerve activity than do city environments', after a 30-minute forest trip. All of these are invaluable for sleep. And another study into the psychological benefits of forest bathing by a team of Japanese researchers concluded that forests are an effective antidote for those with acute emotions, especially those suffering from chronic stress.

Urbanites without a forest in sight can take a walk in a park, which is said to be almost as good as a forest bath for relieving stress, cutting cortisol levels and off-setting the negative build-up that comes with city life. Gardening and tending an allotment also bring the anti-stress, pro-well-being pluses of being outside and surrounded by nature, partly thanks to the biophilia hypothesis, which argues that humans benefit from being close to nature. I always breathe deeply whenever there are trees around, conscious that this is giving my immune system a real boost and bringing my cortisol levels down, which will help me to sleep even better that night.

Keep 'em coming

Have you still got a slight knot in your stomach? Another simple body hack to counter stress is to strike a two-minute power pose – initiating the postural-feedback effect – to send your brain a different message. The postural-feedback effect has had its share of controversy, but it stood up under a 54-study analysis published in 2018, which was carried out to fight back against detractors. The idea was first put forward by professor and social psychologist Amy Cuddy as part of her fake-it-till-you-make-it strategy in her TED Talk 'Your Body Language May Shape Who You Are'.

Here Cuddy argues that just two minutes of power posing before a situation you see as a social threat, or one where you're going to be judged, can increase real power – especially, presumably, if stress or lack of confidence is making you scrunch up into the tiniest ball. It's a tactic that could also be useful for new social or work situations, because first impressions, whether faked or not, have been proven to count, influencing, for example, whether or not you are seen as having leadership qualities. This small intervention, as with Professor Wood Brooks's 'I am excited' experiment, looked at in the previous chapter, shows that we can quickly alter our emotions, behaviour and our reality for the better.

Power posing always makes me smile, and at the very least, it will stop you slumping and sending negative signals to your brain. Hands on hips, legs astride (Wonder Woman), or punching the sky, as if you've just crossed a finish line. I recommend it to my children before exams. And I've used it myself, occasionally. The fact that it feels faintly ridiculous is a mood-boosting game-changer in itself.

Quick cortisol-busters to add to your tool box include:

- Clench your right fist, or squeeze a rubber ball or a tennis ball in your right hand for a few minutes. By engaging these muscles you also activate the left frontal lobe of the brain, which increases feelings of can-do confidence.
- Grip a pen between your teeth for a fake smile. This, too, will trick your body into creating upbeat hormones and emotions that will make you feel happier.
- Breathe deep. Freeze rollercoaster thoughts for a moment and stop shallow breathing – even for a minute or two – as breathing exercises can act as a mini meditation, calming down the central nervous system.

The vagus nerve and deep breathing

Taking deep, slow breaths to calm down is not a new idea, but understand and visualise what it's doing for your body (as a biology-based suggestion), and you can give it extra impact, as practised by Professor Whorwell and Dr Hasan, and which I experienced first-hand back in Chapter 1. Deep breathing not only slows the heart rate, which speeds up with stress, but it also activates the power-wielding vagus nerve, which runs between the brain and body carrying all-important messages to and fro in its role as the main communication highway in the mind–body loop.

The vagus nerve stretches from gut to tongue, vocal cords and brain, via heart, lungs and other organs, and is responsible for controlling our rest-and-digest response. In other words, it calms us down when activated because it is central to the parasympathetic nervous system (PNS), which helps to prepare us for sleep. In contrast, when we're stressed, the sympathetic nervous system (SNS) takes over to action our fight-or-flight process. If the SNS is overactive, this upsets the body's circadian rhythm, which will then block a good night's sleep.

Doctors can stimulate the vagus nerve directly in a hospital environment by using electrical pulses to change the brain's electrical activity and can treat depression, epilepsy and, recently, to bring more than a flicker of consciousness to a patient who had been in a vegetative state for 15 years. If you're just looking to calm down a bit, and you want to get the vagus nerve to send an 'I am calm and not at all stressed' message to brain and body, slow, deep breathing is an effective way to stir it into life (as is humming, splashing cold water on your face or balancing your gut bacteria – more on this later). These methods will mobilise the vagus nerve to release fewer stress signals, and make the heart beat more slowly, so that you can stop stress chemicals from gathering strength during the day and, therefore, sleep more easily at night.

A DIY detox

Deep (diaphragmatic) breathing is not the shallow breathing that hovers below the Adam's apple in the upper chest that we often fall into when we go about our day-to-day activities or exercise, and especially when we're stressed. It's the sort of breathing that pulls air in deeply, making the chest rise and the stomach swell. Deep breathing, typically associated with meditation, not only cuts stress and cortisol levels but it also increases melatonin levels. And aside from being the sleepy hormone, melatonin is a major antioxidant in its own right, in contrast to cortisol, which curbs antioxidant activity. (Antioxidants are molecules that can protect the body from the damaging effects of oxidation and rampaging free radicals. Free radicals are molecules with unpaired electrons, meaning they are on the look-out for electrons to steal from other molecules, at the other molecule's expense. They are a by-product of the

body's metabolic process and they also come about
due to external factors such as pollution, cigarette
smoke, X-rays and some pesticides. Free radicals
and oxidants – those molecules that have already
stolen electrons – can damage the body's cells,
and contribute to a number of long-term health
issues, which is why we need a healthy balance
of antioxidants to off-set them and to disarm free
radicals before they get destructive.)

Cortisol also suppresses your immune system, whereas melatonin
boosts it, so a few well-paced deep breaths here and there, or even
a mini meditation, suddenly seem worth a whole lot more. Also, by
reducing your breaths to just three a minute, you can increase your
slower brainwave frequencies – that is, your alpha and theta brainwaves, as explained on page 50.

One chunk or two?

We might pride ourselves on being able to divide our concentration
every which way, but scientists have shown that the brain struggles
with requests for split-screen attention, and when our primary task is
a tricky one, our performance takes a hit, while our stress chemicals
soar, leaving us in a wound-up state that can hang around well after
lights-out.

It doesn't take much to set off our in-built fight-or-flight mode,
and the cortisol stress spike that goes with it, and trying to simultaneously firefight too many disparate demands will do it. But 'chunking'
can help. The idea behind chunking is that by grouping numbers,
information or jobs together, we've got a better chance of remembering the information or dealing with jobs in the most efficient way

possible, and it harks back to George Miller's ground-breaking paper 'The magical number seven' (1955). Miller's key finding was that our short-term memory can only store between five and nine things at a time – seven plus or minus two – before it loses track, but chunking things together allows us to remember things more easily. Likewise, our brain is more able to store numbers that have been broken down into sections, which is why we fragment phone and pin numbers into a rhythm that we can easily recall.

To-do lists

Working with this theory of what keeps the brain happy (and therefore less stressed), chunking similar jobs together makes for the most efficient time management, allowing us to burn through one block of tasks as quickly as possible before turning to another chunk. A realistic to-do list can also help with this.

I have accumulated way too many lists over the years. But I still make more. There are the digital ones: today/tonight, today/tomorrow, now-ish/whenever (which stops me from getting to-do list fatigue, or any twinges of guilt from staring at to-dos that I don't have the time or the inclination to do), lockdown, personal, work, birthdays/presents, books and films. I also have a list of top to-dos in a green desktop sticky note (which I tend to forget about), and a today/this week one that's generally scribbled down on paper.

Given that the brain doesn't like uncertainty but instead works by trying to problem-solve and predict the future, lists are a good way to feel in control and to empty some of the noise inside our heads.

Practical measures, such as chunking, time management, desktop management, realistic schedules that don't overload you, a to-do whenever list to thin out today's list, a de-cluttered work space and time offline, all help to muzzle overwhelming stress triggers and keep us calmer than we might otherwise be. The same applies to cutting yourself some slack by striking through the non-essential chores (those that are unrealistic for today) that are on your list. All of this will leave you with a clearer head so that you're not left running through tomorrow's to-dos once you're in bed.

A mental list of what we *have* had time to do in the day, rather than berating ourselves for what we *haven't* had time to do, is a better way of looking at things, too. Also, we shouldn't forget to give ourselves plenty of rewards, even if it is just a tick next to a job done, or a 'Well done me', to help bank those positive memories with all the positive emotions and chemicals that go with them.

A word in your shell-like ...

'Tonight, as soon as I decide to go to bed, my sense of the realisation of bedtime will be followed by strong and sustained action throughout my system, which will prepare me for sleep'. This is the opener to Waters' short sleep script that I used to listen to religiously every day at around 5pm when sorting out my sleep. Just listening to it now makes me feel instantly relaxed, reassured and in control, as a sleep script is something that can help us to unwind, as well as to initiate new sleep habits: a stress-buster, suggestion and a sleep-habit cue all rolled into one.

Listening to a sleep script also gives us a welcome pause in the day that buttresses all the other sleep-inducing changes that we're making, and at the same time presenting our brain with a very clear message as to where we are in our sleep countdown. In Chapter 9 we'll be looking more closely at how sleep scripts work, with three different ones for you to choose from.

If you're *still* feeling slightly wired, however, as bedtime approaches – with your mind in hyperdrive rather than slowing down – or if you have a tendency to mull things over in bed, you can always give yourself an armchair offload in a dimly lit room (but not your bedroom). You'll empty that chatter so that you don't carry it off to bed with you, and it schedules time, if needed, to think through tomorrow's timetable as well as any problems or worries, or pleasant things that you want to think about. You can also write an action list, come up with solutions (which your mind will consider while you're sleeping) or have a mindful moment to clear those I'm-awake-and-alert thoughts out of your head.

Stress, worry, anxiety and the rest make terrible bedmates with their stay-awake stress chemicals and their unpleasant physical sensations. But by keeping them in check, looking at them in a different light or disarming them completely, our sleep drive and sleep-inducing neurons can get the elbow room they need so that we can sleep easily and wake recharged.

Having this collection of stress-busting tactics to fall back on has been a real revelation, helping to calm my days, boost my overall well-being and keep my stress levels under control. As a result, I'm not overwhelmed with cortisol at night and my mind is not in overdrive, hyper-aroused and set to spend hours and hours thinking. Instead, I have the chemical balance I need to unwind and sleep deeply as I move through the evening and into the night.

---

4 top tips

1. See stress as enhancing, not debilitating.
2. Switch gripes for gratitudes.
3. Read a book and cut stress by up to 68 per cent.
4. Squeeze a ball in your right hand for can-do confidence.

Chapter 7

The Invisible Rollercoaster – What and When We Eat Matters

A high-calorie shake can make us lose weight, and a late-night snack can help us go to sleep.

Émile Coué had such a sweet tooth that he had only a few teeth left by middle age, and apart from telling his patients to chew their food really well to help with digestion and their gut, food barely gets a mention in his books. Healthy eating was clearly not a top priority a century ago compared to today, when our relationship with food can border on the obsessive, and the benefits of a healthy diet are endlessly discussed.

Having said that, many of us skip breakfast at times. We grab a sandwich for lunch, devour an all-your-nutrients-in-one-go late-night dinner, and pepper the day with high-energy snacks and drinks – all thanks to the go-go-go nature of today. But this top-heavy eating, with sugar-shots to keep us going, comes at a cost. If our eating habits are out of whack with our central body clock and the light and dark going on outdoors, this will quickly undermine our sleep–wake cycle.

'Diet and sleep are connected in a number of different ways,' Dr Eugene Chang tells me. Dr Chang is a gastroenterologist and an expert in gut microbes at the University of Chicago. 'If your gut clock is messed up, your body clock will be messed up and vice versa. They go hand in hand. They talk to each other all the time.'

The optimum time for eating

Chrononutrition – the ideal time to eat certain foods – makes perfect sense and ties in with everything that Dr Chang has observed. Just as light anchors our main biological clock, the timing and content of meals help to anchor the other peripheral clocks that regulate our body's metabolism (the chemical reactions needed to keep the body functioning). And the two systems need to work hand in hand.

For this to happen, the general consensus is that breakfast should be eaten within two hours of waking, followed by a nutritious, sit-down lunch (a short lunch will do) and an early-ish dinner (7–8pm, if you're going to bed at 11pm), with a late-night snack no later than 30 minutes before bed, if needed.

Regular, balanced meals are worth prioritising because they stop us from impulse eating for a quick energy hit, and they help us avoid food cravings and energy lows. If we can include foods rich in the amino acid tryptophan (found in protein-based foods), this will give us the ingredient we need to create the happy hormone serotonin, which is essential to create sleep-inducing melatonin.

We also need to keep our gut life healthy if we want to regulate our sleep–wake patterns, according to Dr Chang. And the high-calorie Western-type diet that's evolved around fast food, with high levels of sugar and salt, seriously works against this.

In a study carried out by Dr Chang into the gut life of mice, he discovered that when the mice in his care were fed a healthy, balanced diet – Mediterranean style – the gut's community of micro-organisms (microbiome) had a distinct rhythm of its own, with 20 per cent of microbes 'oscillating' at night, meaning that their circadian rhythms were nicely balanced.

When the mice were put on a high-fat, high-calorie Western-type diet, however, these microbes stopped oscillating, upsetting the circadian rhythm of the mice, making them put on weight and at the same time changing both their behaviour and their sleep patterns.

I now try to have a more nutritious breakfast than I used to, even if it only comes down to having a handful of nuts, a small bowl of porridge (a good mix of carbohydrates, protein and fibre) and a piece of fruit, or eggs, or avocado on wholegrain toast, with tea. And although I can't say that I breakfast like a king, lunch like a prince and dine like a pauper, as we're often urged to do, because my daily routine doesn't allow for this, I am packing more nutrients into breakfast and lunch than before, followed by an early evening meal, which gives me time to digest it before bed. I also pay attention to the fact that I'm eating so that I don't blink to find my plate bare, having blindly eaten on autopilot. Mindful eating, if you like, which slows down the whole process, gives your brain time to notice when your stomach's full, so that you don't end up overeating.

'When it comes to sleep and food, a lot of it is about routine, timing and planning, so not letting yourself get overly hungry so that you're craving something,' nutritionist Samantha Perkins tells me. She adds:

> It's about *how* you eat, rather than what you're eating. Obviously eating sugary foods before you go to sleep isn't brilliant, because you end up with a sugar spike, and if you miss your evening meal, you're going to get a sugar low. This makes you want to eat a lot of sugary things. Scheduling in a bedtime snack – something like a glass of milk and an oatcake or a banana – rather than having something on impulse would be perfect, because that would top up your sugar levels, give you a bit of energy and make it easier to sleep, because you won't be hungry, and you will be less likely to wake up hungry in the night.

Nothing can be taken in isolation when it comes to the workings of the body, our sleep and health in general, as scientists are increasingly proving. A disrupted feeding rhythm (meal times) messes with all the other body rhythms that are taking place on a daily basis, not just the central night-and-day clock (the SCN in the brain's hypothalamus), but also the rise and fall of that sleepy hormone, melatonin, that peaks at night and melts away in the morning. The rhythms of gut bacteria, body temperature, the 'I'm hungry' hormone, ghrelin, and the 'I'm-full' hormone, leptin, are all connected.

If we eat roughly at the same time each day, however, those molecular body clocks that prepare us for what's lying ahead will be ready and waiting, and hungry or sleepy on cue. But if we feed erratically and late into the evening, when our body should be fasting in its feast–fast cycle, our circadian clocks will be left in a state of confusion with sugar highs and lows in all the wrong places.

That other mind–body loop

Suggestion works by using the mind–body loop, but it's also helped along by the gut–brain axis and the vagus nerve. This is the longest nerve to come out of the brain, and it runs between the brain and the gut, wandering ('vagus' means wandering) via most of the body's major organs along the way, making sure that every part of the body is in cross-communication. The gut talks to the brain. And the brain talks to the gut, making our gut life powerful enough to influence all-round health, moods, stress levels, pain, circadian clocks and sleep.

This means that if our gut is full of sleep-friendly food, our vagus nerve will carry the right messages to our brain. Add to this the fact that 80–90-plus per cent of the happy hormone serotonin is synthesised in the gut, and it seems that we should all have a list of the top ten tryptophan foods needed to do this magnetically welded to our fridge (see the box on the following page).

Tryptophan depletion has also been linked to poor attention and memory, plus anxiety and depression, which can set off insomnia, whereas the feel-good serotonin that comes out of it is known to boost moods, improve memory and help with sleep. A deficiency in serotonin disrupts the sleep–wake cycles, among other things.

GABA is the stress-reliever and shut-down chemical messenger that's produced in the brain and goes to work to reduce activity in the brain and calm our central nervous system so that we can go to sleep. We can find it in foods such as spinach, kale, broccoli, beans, oats, wheat, barley, rice and chestnuts, plus fermented foods such as kimchi.

If you think of the body as a carefully balanced eco-system, where everything is interconnected, it stands to reason that everything you eat, or do, is going to have a knock-on effect on you as a whole: for example, a controlled experiment carried out by a team of Spanish researchers, led by Rafael Bravo, where participants ate tryptophan-enriched cereal at breakfast and dinner for a week (providing three times the tryptophan dose in a standard bowl of cereal) found that the tryptophan-laden cereals 'increased sleep efficiency, actual sleep time, immobile time, and decreased total nocturnal activity, sleep fragmentation index, and sleep latency' (the time it takes to fall asleep), and concluded that tryptophan 'may be useful as a chrononutrition tool for alterations in the sleep/wake cycle', particularly for the elderly, as the serotonin and melatonin rhythms weaken with age.

Tryptophan hero foods

Tryptophan is an essential amino acid, which we need to create the feel-good hormone serotonin, which in turn is needed to create the sleep-inducing hormone melatonin. Tryptophan foods include any food high in protein; that is, all animal products, such as meat, fish, turkey/poultry, eggs, milk, cheese and yogurt, and plant foods high in protein, such as oats (which is why a bowl of oats makes the perfect late-night snack), nuts, chickpeas, sunflower/pumpkin seeds, soya, beans and lentils.

If your bacteria are happy ...

Probiotics are live bacteria that are good for the gut; prebiotics are the foods that feed live bacteria in the gut and they have been found to buffer against stress and improve sleep. These are not the same thing as the probiotics that you can buy as a small capsule or a yoghurt-style drink containing billions of good bacteria. Although probiotics initially produce a dramatic spike in the gut's good bacteria, they are fragile and easily destroyed in the intestinal tract.

Prebiotic foods, on the other hand, are not fragile, and once in the gut they provide food for the gut's existing good bacteria. Good examples are: raw cabbage, apples, bananas, asparagus, onions, leeks, garlic, Jerusalem artichokes, dandelion greens/roots, cooked bran, beans, legumes (lentils, chickpeas and green peas), root vegetables (sweet potatoes, squash, wild yams, jicama, beetroot, carrots, turnips, parsnips), baked wheat flour, fermented foods (such as yogurt, kimchi and sauerkraut), plus miso soup, dark chocolate and pickles. A varied, prebiotic-rich diet increases your gut microbes, which is the ideal gut life for all of us.

Stress, in contrast to prebiotics, is the enemy of good bacteria (whereas exercise is the opposite), impacting the gut's microbiota as well as being one of the biggest disrupters of sleep. Promising early research suggests, however, that following a bout of stress, prebiotics can restore balance to the gut and daily rhythms and can help to improve sleep.

The power that gut microbes have over moods and general health is only just starting to be fully appreciated; for example, the billions of healthy good bacteria that come out of eating prebiotics are also believed to ease pain, potentially providing a non-pharmaceutical answer for those who can't sleep because of it, such as those with fibromyalgia, who, it transpires, have an overgrowth of bad bacteria in their guts.

Stop. Eat. Sleep

Waters was a creature of habit, when it came to food. Regular meals and a big English roast on Sunday, with wine and whisky, structured his week. Today, when food is often reduced to the status of a fuel that we barely stop to register, this lack of a foodie structure can work against us on a number of levels: it can disrupt our sleep routine and our body clocks, take away the perfect opportunity for a pause (for stress spikes to drop), and it makes us put on weight.

'It's about giving your body the time to sit and stop,' says Perkins, when we meet to discuss the impact of diet on sleep. 'If you set regular meals and give yourself time to actually sit down, relax, enjoy your meal and make yourself emotionally and psychologically feel like you've had a meal, and you do that three times a day, then you feel more in control of your food intake. It is easy to think we eat less when we don't have proper meals but we pick and snack instead, as we don't really register it.' And picking and snacking tends to be high-fat, high-calorie stop-gaps that we're drawn to as a fast-acting pick-me-up to stop us flagging.

We have to be realistic, of course. Few of us have time to cook from scratch for every meal or do anything fancy for breakfast, but energy giving, sleep-friendly meals can be quick and easy. A balanced breakfast could be a glass of water (as the body needs to rehydrate in the morning) followed by a bowl of porridge, or eggs, hummus, avocado, tuna mayo and a piece of fruit.

Lunch and dinner need to include, protein, vitamins, a small amount of fats (because some vitamins, such as vitamin D, are fat soluble), and carbohydrates, ideally slow-release carbohydrates. (These are carbohydrates that release their sugar slowly thereby avoiding rises and dips in blood sugar. Slow-release carbohydrates include oats, wholegrain pasta, longer-grain rice, lentils/beans, sweet potato and wholegrain foods). Healthy daytime snacks include fruit, nuts and seeds. Your evening meal could just be pasta, a ready-made sauce, with some cheese and vegetables, and a banana for a bedtime snack, says Perkins. White bread, white potatoes and short-grain white rice are best avoided in the evening in favour of the low-glycaemic-index carbohydrates given above, as these will release sugar slowly into the blood over the next few hours. Sugar highs followed by a sugar dip from refined foods such as white bread will have you reaching for more sugar, which you don't want just before bed.

It's useful to be aware of how food – what we eat and when – affects our sleep, and although I don't overthink all of this, I keep it in mind, leaning towards quick and tasty meals with plenty of prebiotics and tryptophan (protein-based) foods to help me sleep.

If you want to be even more focused on this, there are also functional foods that are said to carry a sleep-promoting punch. These include: whole grains, kiwi fruit, cherries (tart cherry juice ups melatonin, as cherries are a natural source of melatonin), maca, walnuts, lettuce (with hypnotic qualities that were compared to diazepam in one study) and milk, with barley grass powder (packed with GABA, calcium, potassium and tryptophan) seen as sitting on top of the heap, although research into the links between food and sleep still has a way to go.

Avoiding carbohydrates altogether in the evening, as some do, is misguided, says Perkins, because if you don't have those low-glycaemic-index carbohydrates releasing sugar into your blood slowly, 'You're going to get hungry and you're going to have that sugar dip, which means that you're more likely to eat later on in the evening and snack on sugary things, because you're body's going, "I need sugar."'

What we do need to avoid for the best sleep possible are stimulants – of any kind. Whether that's a huge, or high-sugar, late-evening meal, caffeine (which will hang around in your system for hours), chocolate and other high-sugar treats, nicotine or alcohol. Alcohol – an extremely popular self-prescribed sleeping pill – is in fact no good for sleep. Yes, it will knock you out faster, but while your initial deep sleep will be deeper, the second half of the night will go to seed, and you'll likely wake up as your body tries to process the alcohol. Your REM/dream sleep will also suffer.

A single, or a double?

The caffeine hit we get with tea, coffee and other caffeinated drinks has a half-life; that is to say, its strength is roughly halved every 4–6 hours. If you have a caffeinated drink at 10am, for example, after 4–6 hours it will be half its original strength, then 4–6 hours after that a quarter, and so it goes on. At worst there'll still be one-quarter of it left in your system at 10 o'clock at night, at best about one-eighth. We all have different thresholds on this, although some people can sleep after the strongest coffee, it will still impact their sleep, but your ideal caffeine cut-off can be found with a bit of experimentation.

Eat late. Gain weight

If you go for a late, biggest-meal-of-the-day option come evening, you pull apart your central and peripheral body clocks, which are trying to work together to keep your sleep drive on the straight and narrow. What's more, your body is flooded with all those nutrients, but all you've got planned for the evening is a movie or some more desk-bound work before lights-out. With no time to burn it off, a late-night refuel will keep the body stimulated when what it wants to be doing is powering down, ready for bed. Plus, any excessive energy intake at night will turn to fat, according to Dr Chang.

'It's all about time,' says Dr Chang. 'If you're eating and consuming calories at a time when your body is shut down and saying it needs to store that energy, it's not going to burn that energy, it's going to store it as fat.' The reason for this, he says, is that our daily rhythms organise us to 'burn energy during the daytime when we're active and foraging for food and at night-time they turn the switch off and tell our body to rest, store energy and get ready for the next day'.

It's a self-perpetuating circle when it comes to food, sleeplessness and putting on weight. Nutrient-heavy evenings, inadequate tryptophan and erratic eating disconnect the gut from the sleep–wake cycle, leading to poor sleep. Too little sleep then leaves the body short on the 'I'm not hungry/I'm full' leptin hormone, but loaded with 'I can't eat enough to fill me up' ghrelin. The knock-on exhaustion makes us even more likely to reach for extra high-calorie snacks to keep us going – as does stress, because foods taste less sweet when we're stressed, making us eat more to satisfy that sweet-tooth craving.

Obesity and being overweight are also linked to snoring, which leaves you feeling more tired in the day, and, more seriously, to obstructive sleep apnoea (OSA). In this condition sleepers temporarily stop breathing as a result of relaxed throat muscles that block the body's airways. This is followed by a large gasp as they suck in air (a potentially fatal condition that should be brought to the attention of your doctor asap).

Obesity is also connected to type-2 diabetes, where the pancreas and liver can stop working properly, and the pancreas stops producing enough insulin to keep glucose moving out of the blood and into the body's cells. This leads to a rise in blood sugar levels (a precursor to type-2 diabetes). Both obesity and lack of sleep have also been linked to insulin resistance. Diet and improved sleep can help to tackle all these, with a low-calorie, type-2 diabetes reversal diet seeing remission in 90 per cent of patients.

A team of researchers led by Jean-Phillipe Chaput found that the 'average weight gain of short-duration sleepers [5–6 hours] is 88 per cent more than the weight gain of average-duration sleepers [7–8 hours]'. While the six-year Quebec Family study found 'long-duration sleepers' (9–10 hours) also gain significant weight and fat, similar to the short-duration sleepers, suggesting that there's a sweet spot to be reached in the middle.

The take-away from all this being that regular meals, and smaller, early evening Mediterranean dinners, can help us to get the sleep we need, and lose weight in the process. Besides, pre-bedtime snacks are still on the menu. In fact, a low-calorie (less than 200 kcals) late-night snack, 90 minutes after a light early evening meal, has been put forward as an effective way to lose weight, improve muscle strength and help with sleep. Researchers found that those who ate a small bowl of oat-based cereal (as oats are high in tryptophan) with low-fat milk 30 minutes before bed for four weeks ate fewer calories each day and evening and lost a small amount of weight, which was put down to eating less at night in the knowledge that a snack was on the cards later.

More calories, please

The placebo diet is something that Coué, arguably the father of placebo, and Waters would both have been fascinated by, although, no doubt, not that surprised by. The discovery that it's not only the calories we eat that make us put on weight, or feel hungry or full, but what we *believe* about the food that we're putting into our mouths – the Coué and Waters' power of suggestion is at work once again here.

Take the milkshake experiment led by Alia Crum, assistant professor of psychology and director of the Mind and Body Lab at Stanford University, which overturns everything we thought we knew about our relationship with food, calories and weight gain.

Here, two milkshakes were served up on different days to a group of willing milkshake drinkers. Milkshake 1, the 'Indulgence' at 620 calories per serving, was high in saturated fat (91 per cent), cholesterol (39 per cent) and sodium (19 per cent). It was labelled 'Decadence you deserve' over a picture of a mountain of ice cream topped with sprinkles and described as 'rich, creamy and irresistibly satisfying' – enough to add an extra inch at a glance. Milkshake 2, the 'Sensi-Shake', in stark contrast offered 'Guilt-free satisfaction for the health-conscious buyer', a 'sensible' choice with 0 per cent fat, zero sugar and only 140 calories per serving, alongside an image of an 'I'm not at all indulgent' vanilla flower.

The Sensi-Shake left drinkers feeling hungry with little change in their 'I'm hungry' ghrelin levels – the hunger hormone – and therefore more than likely to go on a snack-run later. The Indulgence, in sharp contrast, hit the spot, with drinkers experiencing a dramatic drop in their 'I'm hungry' hormones.

The only problem with these results was that the milkshakes were identical, calorie for calorie. It was the drinkers' expectations that influenced the shakes' effects on their bodies. The bitter irony being that those going for the healthy option appeared to harness the nocebo effect – the negative sibling of the placebo effect – that is, the negative *expectation* to still feel hungry as a result of eating low-fat, low-calorie foods.

To make matters even worse for those trying to be good, the higher your 'I'm hungry' hormones are, the more your body will store fat. The way that works is that the longer we don't eat, the higher our ghrelin levels go, sending a clear message to the brain to go and find some food. Meanwhile, the body will slow down its metabolism to store energy in case there's a food shortage out there, which means that with ghrelin levels almost unchanged you're not burning off that low-calorie milkshake you've just had.

The bottom line is that the Sensi-Shake did not make hunger pangs plummet, the researchers concluded, because we don't *expect* diet foods to be as satisfying as high-calorie ones, given their association with self-denial and the rest.

Packaging is clever and, as with all adverts, it makes good use of direct suggestions – the end result of carefully planned marketing strategies, where key words and ingredients are put centre stage, to pull the shopper in. Keeping the Sensi-Shake and the Indulgence

milkshakes in mind, which both used deliberately misleading suggestion in their packaging and their ingredients, we might be better off
going for something we see as a treat, or as Crum, et al., argue, train
ourselves to savour every bite and eat with an indulgent mindset:
'Yum, this plain cracker is *so* delicious' and watch our appetites fall,
while our fat-burning metabolism fires up and our body's 'I'll keep
that in the larder for later' survival instinct steps back.

Eat with an indulgent mindset and you can help yourself to not eat
stimulating, calorific snacks too close to bedtime and to feel full on
less, speed up your metabolism and stop yourself feeling hungry when
you want to sleep.

Cupboard love

If you're looking for ways to lift your mood via your stomach, to work
alongside suggestion, emotional swaps or stress-busting techniques,
Perkins recommends folate and selenium supplements. (Selenium can
also be found in nuts, seeds, meat and fish.) For those of us not getting
enough sunshine during the winter months, a vitamin D supplement
can make up the loss, while B vitamins release energy from carbohydrates, so they can help to counteract tiredness.

'In terms of supplements, if someone wasn't confident that they
were eating a really good balanced diet, a multivitamin is the best
thing. You want to avoid taking big doses of anything,' says Perkins.
And it's worth getting your doctor to check that you haven't got any
major deficiencies, as a lack of magnesium, omega-3, vitamin D and
vitamin C, for example, have all been linked to disrupted or third-
rate sleep.

Valerian is a popular herbal sleep aid and melatonin has been used
for years in the US to help with sleep, particularly by those suffering
from jet lag, with research ongoing into their effectiveness or how they
might work when combined with other supplements. Magnesium
salts, pills and sprays are also said to help with sleep, if you're deficient

in magnesium. I have tried all three in the past, plus endless sleepy teas from the local health shop, but in such an ad hoc way that I can't vouch for any of them. (Studies suggest that melatonin and magnesium need longer than I gave them to have any major effect, with one 2019 study finding that a particular magnesium, melatonin and vitamin B complex needed to be taken for three months for sleepers to feel the benefits – and the jury is out on whether valerian helps.) Although I seem to remember that they did help me a bit, at the very least on a placebo level I guess, it wasn't enough to give me a reliable and regular sleep–wake pattern or to stop me needing prescription sleeping pills when things got out of control.

Cannabidiol (CBD), a component of cannabis that doesn't come with a high, and which is legal in America, has different restrictions in Europe depending on where you live, and L-theanine, found in tea leaves, are two natural supplements that have had a lot of press, with a growing number of studies into their relaxing and sleep-promoting properties. CBD has been found to be effective for reducing anxiety and pain, while L-theanine has been shown to reduce the amount of time it takes to get to sleep and increase the amount of time spent asleep, when combined with GABA.

Precision medicine is also on the horizon, says Dr Chang, where the individual's unique gut life could be helped to reduce the production of bad molecules and upgrade the production of good molecules, bypassing the gut microbiome and diet altogether (so we can all have our cake and eat it). 'What you're talking about are interventions that are very, very practical,' Dr Chang tells me, 'that is, people take these good molecules that promote leanness, less stress and sleep in a capsule, like a vitamin, along with their breakfast. I think that's the future.'

All that sounds very sci-fi. For now, though, it appears that our best bet is a Mediterranean-type diet, as much as possible, rich in fruit, vegetables, legumes (beans, peas and lentils), nuts, grains, beans, cereals, fish, starchy foods, and unsaturated fats, such as olive oil, and plenty of water (although not just before bed, if you want uninterrupted sleep), with lots of tryptophan foods as listed on pages 145–146, and an indulgent mindset when we eat certain foods. And if we can give ourselves a good food routine, and keep stimulating, fast-release treat foods for earlier in the day, we can avoid sugar peaks and troughs too close to bedtime, which will mess with our rhythms, disrupt our sleep and make it too easy to confuse tiredness, thirst or a lack of energy with hunger. Instead of eating more food the more tired we get, we can replace high-calorie cravings post evening dinner with a tryptophan snack and an earlier night.

4 top tips

1. Keep regular(ish) mealtimes – three times a day.
2. Pack your diet with tryptophan-rich foods, for maximum serotonin and melatonin.
3. Eat a Mediterranean diet for an even sleep–wake cycle.
4. Eat low-calorie late-night snacks no less than 30 minutes before bed.

Chapter 8

Feeling Flush

The silent taboo: sleep wreckers that depend on where in
the world women live – and how women and men can turn
back the clock of time.

Hot, bloated, uncomfortable, in pain … when it comes to sleep,
women have extra obstacles thrown at them, whether that's the fluctuating heat or cramps of the monthly menstrual cycle or, generally
more disruptive, the hot flushes, night sweats, anxiety and insomnia
that can come with peri-menopause (the period before menopause)
and menopause, which can last for decades. And while most people are
aware of the discomfort and inconvenience of periods, menopause is
largely off-radar: a taboo subject that's barely discussed, despite it being
a natural body change that affects half the global population, with the
number of postmenopausal women set to reach 1.1 billion by 2025.
The thing that doesn't add up at first glance is that women can suffer
from specific menopausal symptoms in some cultures, while in others
they don't – cultural suggestions being *that* powerful, once again.

It doesn't help that both these biological realities are often the butt of jokes, misinformation or, as is often the case with menopause, little information at all in the Western world. Without hard facts and an understanding of what's going on beneath your skin, how is it possible to be prepared, know what to do or not to be taken by surprise? Because unless women are prepped for their physical future so that body changes can be minimised and managed, their day-to-day reality and quality of life can take a major hit, leaving their sleep in tatters and them feeling drained and much, much older than they really are. And age, it turns out, is also at the mercy of suggestion and expectations, with those women who live in societies where youth is lauded and old age lamented apparently experiencing much worse menopausal symptoms as a result.

The incubator within

More than 85 per cent of menstruating women suffer at least one period symptom every month: headaches, cramps, tender breasts, depression, anxiety, nausea, diarrhoea, bloating, constipation and mood swings. So it's little wonder that one or more of these will regularly disrupt their sleep. On top of this, there's another, less well-known culprit that can interfere with your sleep. And that's the hormone progesterone. To put it simply, oestrogen cools us down, while progesterone heats us up, and during the second half of the menstrual cycle (post ovulation) there's a progesterone spike, meaning that we get more body heat. It's thought that the extra heat might be needed to develop the egg, much like an incubator. But given that we need our body temperature to drop one or two degrees at night to have undisturbed sleep, this can obviously lead to restless nights.

Thankfully the body's sleep–wake rhythm is generally able to adjust itself around these monthly oscillations, with only one in ten women saying that sleep problems impact their day, in a survey by the National Sleep Foundation; however, 30 per cent did say that their sleep is disturbed during their period, with 23 per cent noticing that they had more disturbed sleep in the week before menstruation and 50 per cent saying that they were likely to be in a bad mood if they were sleepy during the day. Who hasn't heard a joke about PMS (premenstrual syndrome) and the moods that come with this? If we can improve our sleep, however, we can obviously soften those stereo-typical PMS markers.

For those knock-out stomach cramps, or dull aches, a hot water bottle, electric heat pads or on-the-go wraps, hugged closely, are tried-and-tested favourites, and caffeine-free pain relief is another option come night. But you could also try keeping a sleep diary for a couple of months to see what's happening with your sleep and when it is disturbed. If it's heat waking you up in the night in the second half of your cycle, at least you'll know what's causing it and that it will soon stop when your progesterone levels drop off. Meanwhile, you can keep your bedroom cool (radiator low or off) and a fan within reach, and sleep with light layers on your bed, ones that are easy to throw aside so that you can get your core body temperature back down to where it needs to be to go back to sleep.

Where's the shame in that?

With menopause, the number of women affected is more dramatic – as is the fallout. And it's the night sweats that are said to be keeping most women awake. 'Sleep, as an issue for women going through the peri-menopause and menopause, is huge. Huge. At least half of my patients have an issue with it,' says Dr Mary Jane Minkin, professor in obstetrics, gynaecology and reproductive health at Yale Medical School. Dr Minkin specialises in menopausal health and has an edu-cational website for women and professionals that goes through all the various options that are out there (http://madameovary.com). 'And my peri-menopausal and menopausal patients who have been up night after night, after night are chronically exhausted. How is their mood and their cognitive issues? It is not good,' she tells me.

Up to 90 per cent of menopausal women in the West suffer from hot flushes during the day and night sweats that ruin their sleep. And while the average age for menopause is 51 (a year after your last period), the range is anything from 45 to 55 years, and the lead up to this begins 4–6 years before with sleep problems sometimes starting then and subsequently dragging on and on. Early menopause is officially classified as anything before the age of 45, although it can start much earlier for a number of different reasons, including cancer treatment or surgery to remove the ovaries. I'm not clear when my peri-menopause started, as I wasn't paying it any attention. My body's menstrual cycle had been erratic for years, having gone to the wall immediately after I had my twin boys and never fully recovering after that. I simply assumed that my body had nothing to spare, having grown three babies in a relatively short amount of time, so I just lived with irregular on–off periods until eventually they stopped, earlier than they probably would have done otherwise.

A big problem with how women deal with their menopause, according to experts, is a sense of shame, secrecy and embarrassed silence that often surrounds it, with many women battling on without seeking help or support. I have to hold my hand up and be counted as one who didn't really discuss what I was going through. Why? I'm not altogether sure. I guess it was a combination of not having read up about what was happening inside my body, the physical changes not being that bad, and a slight feeling that it was just 'women's stuff' that others probably wouldn't want to hear about and something that might just go away if I ignored it, which it did. Although night sweats is a graphic description, if anything it falls short of the drenching that can take place, and it is hardly glamorous or something you might always want to share. Night flush – which would be a coy euphemism – might be easier to run with, or discuss. Whatever was at play, I'm not alone. A survey carried out by the British Menopause Society found that 50 per cent of women don't even talk to their doctor about their menopausal symptoms, despite 42 per cent of them saying menopause was worse, or much worse, than they had expected.

Cultural baggage worth losing

Feeling 'old' really doesn't help (for either women *or* men, see below), because the menopause women experience tends to depend on where they live and how ageist that society is, according to Dr Minkin and others, with the severity of symptoms changing according to where they are on the global map; for example, in North America, Europe and Brazil, women can have a hard time of it, whereas in other countries and cultures a woman's menopause can be just a blip on life's landscape: mild, or even something to be celebrated, thanks, it's argued, to different attitudes towards older women and a sense of freedom and status that can come with advancing years.

Whereas hot flushes are top of the list in the West and a major sleep disrupter, Japanese women complain of stiff shoulders, with only 12–20 per cent of Asian women reporting hot flushes; Singaporean women have lower backache and aching muscles and joints more than any other symptom (51 per cent); few Indian women experience the menopause symptoms that we have in the West (one study finding just 34 per cent to have hot flushes/night sweats, and this was largely put down to anxiety, spicy foods, poorer health and more negative beliefs about menopause); and women from Yucatan, Mexico, who are descendants of the Mayans, have few if any complaints and actually look forward to their menopause. In the Philippines, the number-one complaint is achiness. Number two is headaches and number three is hot flushes. In the United States, women suffer achiness, too, but nowhere nearly as badly as they do hot flushes. Why is there this much variety for something you would have thought is universal? Research so far doesn't have a definitive answer as to why menopause symptoms appear to be determined by where women live, although the negative versus positive attitudes to women and age and menopause are seen as key.

'Women with more negative attitudes towards the menopause in general report more symptoms during the menopausal transition,' concluded a review of 13 studies on menopause, led by Ayers. Is this the nocebo effect at play again (in the West), with women's negative associations and expectations affecting their actual experience? It's possible.

'In cultures where the older women are valued and revered, many of the women don't complain of the symptoms,' says Dr Minkin, 'whereas in the United States, particularly, where youth is totally revered, these are horrible symptoms and people will suffer with them. We're not supposed to get old. That's not a glamorous and good thing to do. There are tremendous negative connotations and the image is not favourable. The kind of perception that's there is that people going through menopause are ditzy, crazy ladies. It's not considered glamorous to be a menopausal lady, which is part of the reason we don't talk about it.' Whatever is going on, lifestyle and cultural norms, including what women are comfortable reporting, presumably play a part in the global menopause picture that's emerging.

Young at heart is just the start of it

Studies show that if you tell yourself 'I'm so old' with a grimace and a game-over attitude, you actually make yourself age more quickly. By thinking of yourself as a stereotypical old person – slow, creaky, falling apart at the seams, forgetful and in need of help – what you're doing is creating a self-fulfilling prophecy, with your imagination, self-talk, brain signals and expectations stacked up against you.

In one of many experiments that expose how flexible age can be, carried out by Professor Becca R. Levy, from Yale University, and discussed in her paper 'Mind Matters', a group of older individuals were subliminally exposed to positive words associated with age, flashed up on a computer screen fast enough to allow 'perception without awareness'. Walking speed was measured before and after, and the study found that afterwards participants actually walked faster. Studies also show that those with a more positive take on growing old see themselves as healthier, take more risks, depend less on others and feel less lonely. Elderly Chinese people, who tend to have a positive view about growing old, have better memories than North Americans. Exposure to positive age stereotypes can sharpen the brain, improve memory, tighten up old-vs-young handwriting, give you the will to live, *and* make you live 7½ years longer than others who are less positive about the idea of growing old, Levy and her team have discovered – all of which comes down to suggestion.

In an infamous counter-clockwise experiment in 1979 led by Ellen Langer, professor of psychology at Harvard University, scientists effectively turned back the clock by taking a group of elderly men and putting a spring in their step in a matter of days. The group of eight men, who were all in their seventies, were taken to a retreat in New Hampshire that had been decked out as if it was 1959, down to what was on the black-and-white television and old-time radio.

The men were told to behave as if it was 1959, 20 years earlier than it actually was, and to talk only in the present tense. No mirrors were allowed, just photographs of their younger selves, and they were asked not to talk about *anything* post 1959. Daily discussions were scheduled about 'recent' events such as the previous year's (1958) launch of the first US satellite, *Explorer 1*, or 'recent' books such as Ian Fleming's *Goldfinger*. They listened to the likes of Nat King Cole and watched films such as *Some Like it Hot*.

Langer later wrote that she felt the most important part of the experiment was the fact that the scientists had decided not to make the retreat more elderly friendly. No obstacles had been removed to make it easier for them to get about, as 'lack of obstacles signals incompetence'. The men were left to get themselves and their belongings to their rooms, navigate stairs and sort out what to do if they dropped anything on the floor. Despite the fact that they were used to being helped in countless ways by their families and having their meals served for them, the men very quickly became more independent, serving and clearing their own dishes and generally fending for themselves. Five days later, their physical strength, mental health and cognitive abilities had *all* improved – as had their hearing, memory and eyesight. They even *looked* younger.

All of this makes me think of a friend of a friend who I met in one of those north London pubs that's a real locals' pub. He is someone who's clever, energetic, articulate and interesting, learning Arabic for fun; his wife was at home and he had just popped in for a quick drink to catch up with friends and discuss the news, politics and literature. I was thrown when someone told me he was 84 years old. I would have struggled to put an age on him, but he seemed many years younger than that. His ageless behaviour and conversation made it impossible and completely irrelevant to define him by years.

Langer believes we wrongly associate age with decay, with disastrous results. We are, in fact, simply *changing*, not decaying, she says. And her years of hands-on research suggest that what we're doing is *behaving* 'old' – focusing on and clinging to any perceived physical failings and limitations – because society *expects* this of us. We are showing signs of age that we've been told come with the job title: self-imposed restrictions that don't need to be there, actively encouraged by society and those around us. And most of these signs, needless to say, are negative, with menopause dropped into the middle of all that.

If menopause and age are seen as going together, looking at age and the growing-old process from a more positive standpoint can only help. After all, we can all choose to be perennials now, that is to say, *not* defined by age, but by behaviour, tastes and interests, forever blooming and curious, whatever decade we're in. In which case, menopause can be a 'so what?' sign that the years are passing. And an acceptance of menopause, studies show, makes symptoms less frequent and the whole experience less intense and easier to manage.

Keeping the seesaw steady

Hot flushes, night sweats and other symptoms of menopause are not only apparently made better or worse depending on how your society views older women, but also by a number of other life factors, including how much money you earn, whether you have some form of higher education or not, your body mass index (BMI), whether you smoke, how much alcohol you drink and whether you've had a hysterectomy. If you're ticking too many of these boxes for your liking, take heart, because a 2018 study supported by the National Institutes of Health ('Sleep problems during the menopausal transition') argued that a woman's experience of the menopause could be hugely improved if it was just *normalised* (in other words, part of her everyday conversation) if mood disorders were proactively dealt with *and* by addressing the issue of sleep.

Easy fixes for a cool sleep

- A really cool bedroom, nightclothes made with light, natural fibres, plus having light layers of natural-fibre bedding that can be thrown off as needed can help to prevent and deal with night sweats.
- Wool mattress toppers are not only great for extra comfort but they are also touted for their ability to disperse body heat and stop your heat from bouncing back at you from your mattress.
- You could also have a fan to cool the bedroom (preferably within reach, so that you're not forced to get out of bed to turn it on) in addition to keeping a window open, filling a hot water bottle with iced water, and having to hand a wet flannel or cold pack (possibly in a small cooler bag with ice block), or other cooling aids that work for you.
- Keep fresh nightclothes to hand so that you can get dry and comfortable fast.

- Cool down quickly by sticking your hands
  and feet out from underneath your bedding.
  This will help to bring down your core body
  temperature quickly.
- Turn your pillow over, then challenge and replace
  any sleep-panic thoughts by saying to yourself,
  'This will pass and I will get enough sleep
  to manage'.
- Do some deep, abdominal breathing throughout,
  and then go back to sleep.

Menopause (from the Greek words for month and pause) is that time in life when women stop having their periods due to a drop in oestrogen as well as progesterone. Their ovaries stop releasing an egg each month, so they're no longer able to get pregnant. Peri-menopause, menopause and post-menopause are parts of a woman's natural ageing process. Some argue that there's a male menopause, too – the andropause – but others argue against this notion, as the testosterone decline is minimal compared to the more sudden oestrogen drop experienced by women.

The body's thermostat (controlled by the hypothalamus) goes slightly haywire during the peri-menopause, menopause and post-menopause thanks to fluctuating hormones and the drop in oestrogen. Previously, oestrogen worked to keep the body's heat on an even keel, but now, with lower oestrogen levels, the body cools itself down by releasing heat via a hot flush. Night sweats are the nocturnal version of this, where sleepers wake up to find themselves soaked in sweat, and it's these broken nights due to waking up hot that women say is the main reason that their sleep falls apart, leaving them exhausted during the day.

If women are able to look at their menopause through a different lens, however, and use practical tactics for any day-to-day symptoms they do experience, they can manage the physical changes that take place and get the sleep they need, allowing them to carry on as usual with their lives.

Mean and moody

Mood swings can, unfortunately, come with the menopause package, with depression a possible side effect, too. And a negative take on growing old is obviously not going to help. Added to this the drop in oestrogen affects how much of the happy serotonin hormone we produce, and with low serotonin come low moods and poor sleep. This is where serotonin boosters come into their own, as discussed in Chapter 6, as well as making sure you have plenty of tryptophan in your diet (see pages 145–146) to maximise how much serotonin you can make and how much melatonin can come out of that.

Exhaustion, irritability, not being able to think straight, temporary forgetfulness and weight gain are also so-called signs of menopause. But these are also what you get if you don't sleep well at night or you are chronically sleep-deprived, as many menopausal women are, which is why Dr Hadine Joffe, at Nash General Hospital, Boston, has conducted studies where, rather than dealing with the hormonal issues, women are just given sleep medication. And the results are positive. 'Indeed,' confirms Dr Minkin, 'they do tend to improve their cognition the next day and feel better. And they feel better mood-wise from just getting a decent night's sleep.'

Being overweight also makes hot flushes that much worse, as the extra weight is thought to trap the heat of a hot flush. Therefore, while exercise will not help your hot flushes in the first instance, the weight loss that comes with this will help in the long term, plus exercise will give your moods another lift. You can also help to counteract mood swings and negativity (which will then improve your sleep and lift your moods) by having a mini re-boot with some scheduled-in me-time for something that you enjoy doing, *every* day – even if you can only manage 5 minutes. By prioritising this for yourself – a run, walk, chat with a friend, time alone, a book-reading session, being outdoors – you give your moods a boost and bring stress down, and with it the inflammatory effect stress has on the body, which will, of course, help to improve your sleep, too.

I would say, looking back, that I was definitely moodier during my peri-menopause and menopause. Snappier. More stressed. More irritable, flat and tearful ... but then again, my sleep was dreadful. And everything feels so much worse and overwhelming when you're chronically sleep deficient. Given what I now know about the menopause and how the experience can be so different depending on where you live, whether you see opportunities diminishing with the years, whether you dread the idea of growing old or not, and what you *expect* to experience physically (given that menopausal symptoms are not universal), I'm inclined to think that a lot of that emotional moodiness was mainly the result of too little sleep (for years), an exhausting family life and possibly a small, menopausal, it's-all-over-now cloud hovering over my head.

In. And. Out

Hot flushes are *very* responsive to the way we breathe. Deep, controlled breathing: breathing in to the count of five and out to the count of five – which brings the number of resting breaths down from 12–20 per minute to just six – is incredibly effective when it comes to subduing hot flushes. In one study, led by Richa Sood MD and published in the journal *Menopause*, women who did this for 15 minutes twice a day saw hot flushes drop by 52 per cent. Other research recommends that you breathe through each flush, as they roll, which probably works better for most, as it is something you can use in the moment and not something else you have to add to your daily to-do list and then feel guilty about not doing.

By switching to deep-paced breathing as you feel a hot flush take hold, you're not only asserting control over the situation (by sending the right signals to the brain via the vagus nerve), you are also refocusing your attention away from the flush and on to the breath. You can also make yourself pay attention to whatever you're doing or is going on around you – anything but the hot flush. It's a distraction technique that should stop you from inadvertently stoking the fire through panic by calming the feelings of lost control and worst-case-scenario self-talk. The mind feeding into the body.

Regular controlled breathing also gives us those pauses we need in the day. It creates a moment to stop doing anything at all apart from following your breath, thereby giving you a chance to decompress for a minute, calm the internal chatter and bring tension and cortisol levels down. It becomes something that's soothing and anchoring, hot flush or not.

The thought-habit challenge

Catastrophic thoughts have to go. Stop and listen to your thoughts the next time a hot flush or night sweat moves in. What are you thinking to yourself? Is it along the lines of: *Oh, No. I'm going red. Everyone's staring at me. How embarrassing. I look so sweaty/unprofessional/unattractive. I can't cope. It's getting worse. I'll never get through this presentation?* If so, these kinds of thoughts need to be shown the door and replaced with positive, fact-based ones, such as: *I'll just breathe through this and it will pass shortly. So what if I look a bit red, people will just think the room is too hot or I've been rushing around. No one's paying attention, or even noticing.*

Negative thoughts that knock your confidence and exaggerate how people are reacting to you are not based on reality. Challenging them and switching them for ones that are kinder *and* fairer is an effective method for reducing anxiety in general. It lets you assert some control over the situation and talk down any rising panic that would otherwise feed into a hot flush, making it worse.

Undermining thoughts can set off anxiety, panic and dispropor-tionate self-consciousness – where what you're doing, without even realising it, is looking for threats or negative signs in others where they don't even exist. The reality is more likely to be that others are oblivious, indifferent (in the nicest possible way), sympathetic or empathetic (they've been there, or know someone who has).

If you are in a public place and think that all eyes are trained on you, remind yourself of those mind-wandering statistics on page 116, and the fact that nearly 50 per cent of those around you are thinking about a problem that's on their mind, a past fixation, a future worry, or what they need to buy/do later, their relationship, their wish-list relationship, and so on. Their world centres on them. Not on you.

Of course, in some situations, you might feel that you can just say you're having a hot flush and then move on. People are sympathetic, so research shows, and besides, the more that menopausal symptoms are normalised, the better it will be for all of us. For one, employers need to appreciate that sometimes the heating might need to be turned down, windows thrown open and fans used to cool the room temperature (and yours).

With night sweats being such a major sleep disrupter for so many women, the biology-based suggestions as I have listed above can help to stop the hot flush from escalating and can speed up its exit so that sleep can soon resume. Think: *Breathing into this will calm my hot flush and make it pass much faster. By sticking out my hands and feet, I can help to bring down my core temperature. Once I cool off a bit, this hot flush will subside and I will go back to sleep.*

Dear diary, today . . .

'Dear diary, today I ate a hot, spicy laksa, followed by several beers in a hot, stuffy room, and the next minute I was as red as a beetroot.' A hot-flush/night-sweats diary is a very practical way to get an overview of what's going on, and to see what might be triggering your hot flushes and night sweats or making them worse. Once you see a pattern, you can remove the triggers. They might be hot drinks, alcohol, hot showers/baths, stress, exercise, rushing around, or negative, catastrophic thoughts that can transform a tepid flush into a burning one.

If you find a hot flush sweeps over you when you move from a cold environment to a hot one, or vice versa, you could give yourself a minute for your core body temperature to adjust before carrying on with whatever you're doing. And there are other things that you can do to reduce the chances of setting off a hot flush such as: taking a warm shower/bath, rather than a hot one; exercising somewhere cool; letting hot drinks cool down slightly before you drink them; reducing caffeine; avoiding/reducing alcoholic drinks and spicy foods; and managing your time better, so that you're not left running from A to B.

Try to find a routine or ritual that works for your flushes, whether during the day or at night – nothing rushed (for example, at night slowly remove a layer, reach out, put the fan on, mop your brow, flip your pillow, sip some water, and go back to sleep'). If you can switch to this routine/ritual, it can give you a greater sense of control and create a habit chunk where your brain knows that the hot flush/night sweat is already on its way out. There's also the preventative action you can take during the day, such as being proactive about reducing your stress levels and factoring in me-time to bring general inflammation down. And then with lots of light layers in place, topped with something that can be swiftly removed – a sweater, poncho, shawl – you can bring your body temperature down, barely missing a beat.

Turning back the clock

With everything we know about the gut–brain loop, it makes sense that different diets will give us a different menopause. But it's surprising, nonetheless, that one can give you fewer hot flushes and another can push back your menopause by more than three years.

On average 75 per cent of women in the West say that they suffer from hot flushes (going up to 90 per cent in some studies) whereas only 12–20 per cent of women are reported to experience them in Japan and

China – a massive difference that's partly put down to the soya in their diet. Soya contains weak plant oestrogens known as isoflavones, and a diet high in soya products – such as soya beans, tofu, soy sauce and miso – which is popular in many Asia–Pacific countries, is said to cut the intensity and frequency of hot flushes. The effects of a soya-based diet are slow to kick in but it has an accumulative effect, and it also protects against cardiovascular diseases and certain cancers (such as breast and prostate).

Magnesium-rich foods, such as dark leafy greens, seeds, beans, fish, whole grains, nuts and yogurt, are also said to help with premenstrual symptoms (PMS and premenstrual migraines) and menopausal ones, including reducing hot flushes by over 50 per cent. Despite this, magnesium deficiency is rife worldwide, particularly in the Western world. If we're magnesium deficient, apart from making hot flushes that much worse, we're also at greater risk of becoming anxious, depressed or more stressed (among other things). Flip this by giving yourself a diet packed with foods high in magnesium and you can help to cut your stress and anxiety levels and, therefore, improve your moods and your sleep – in the same way that lots of tryptophan-laden foods can increase your serotonin 'happy hormone' levels, and, in turn, your sleepy melatonin levels.

There are also herbal supplements for menopause out there, of course, although test results for these are largely mixed. In one study that examined 11 brands of black cohosh (which is said to help reduce hot flushes) manufactured in the United States, two were found not to contain any black cohosh at all and the make-up of the others was variable, according to Dr Minkin; however, she swears by a German brand called Remifemin, which she says *does* work and it is backed up by a number of papers and literature.

If you're nowhere near having your menopause, you could just use your diet to take preventative action, introducing plenty of soya to get ahead of the game, as well as choosing a diet that can delay the start of your menopause and expand your reproductive years. By switching refined pasta and rice with wholegrain versions, increasing your fresh legume intake and the amount of oily fish you eat, you can push back the menopause by quite a few years, according to the UK Women's Cohort Study (UKWCS), which looked at feedback from more than 14,000 women aged 35–69 over a four-year period. With just a daily portion of oily fish it found you can postpone your menopause by 3.3 years, and with fresh legumes (such as fresh or frozen, not dried, edamame, peas and green beans) by nearly a year per daily helping – meaning that if you eat two portions of fresh legumes every day, you can delay your menopause by nearly two years – whereas refined pasta and rice will do the opposite, bringing menopause forward by 1½ years per daily portion. Vitamin B6 and zinc were also linked to a later menopause start date.

Some women, of course, opt for hormone replacement therapy (HRT) to deal with menopause symptoms, and you're best off discussing this with a specialist doctor. If this is not for you, or you're still suffering from hot flushes or night sweats well beyond the menopause, when HRT is less effective and said to be riskier, the options covered earlier – education, conversation, acceptance and some proactive menopause-management tips – have been shown to get results.

Women can maintain or dramatically improve the quality of their life and their sleep from the peri-menopause onwards by challenging any sense of stigma, overturning our negative attitudes towards menopause and age, reducing stress and boosting moods, as well as paced breathing *throughout* hot flushes, fact-based suggestion, a hot-flush/night-sweats diary, a menopause-friendly diet and taking action to avoid triggers.

4 top tips

1. Schedule in daily me-time to relax (however brief).
2. Keep a hot-flush/night-sweats diary.
3. Wear layers that can be easily removed.
4. Use controlled abdominal breathing to manage hot flushes/night sweats.

Chapter 9

Are You Listening Carefully?

This is not *just* a sleep script. It is a pause in your day.
A chemical balancer. A thought-habit moulder.
A sleep-habit cue. A behavioural trigger.

'Tonight, as soon as I decide to go to bed, my sense of the realisation of bedtime will be followed by strong and sustained action throughout my system, which will prepare me for sleep. As I move off to my room, I will commence automatically to relax in mind and body. All the nervous strain and tension of the day will drop away and as I undress and generally prepare for bed, I will be inwardly preparing for rest and sleep even more completely. Thus, I will find myself in bed, restful in mind, functionally restful in body and as this good habit of changing my state every night develops ever more fully, I will obtain ever more complete, full and restful sleep.'

I used to listen to the above very brief sleep script that Waters wrote in 1937, which I recorded for myself on my phone, and I started doing this soon after coming across Waters' segment on insomnia in

So Built We the Wall, which, as you know, set me off on this sleep-science quest.

In Waters' day, scripts were given as a printout, to be read by the patient,and have since been upgraded to a recording. Today, audio scripts are used all the time with cognitive therapy and clinical hypnosis.

A sleep script is a potent sleep-habit cue. What it does, in a daily, drip-drip kind of way, just as Coué's mantra worked on a more general level, is help to re-write the brain's sleep habits and embed positive sleep suggestions until these sleep thought patterns and subsequent behaviours become our reality. And, of course, it's the repetition of these positive sleep suggestions (as discussed in Chapter 4) that gather force every time you listen to them, because what you're doing is helping to build a new sleep habit, layer by layer, to submerge the old habit that you want to get rid of.

I resisted introducing this sleep-script chapter earlier in the book because it's important to have a clear understanding of sleep and to be able to see why and how sleep scripts work in this context for them to be properly effective. You first need to have an idea of the science, clinical hypnosis, habit formation, sleep biology and the physiological changes that can be brought about by words alone. You can't *simply* listen to a sleep script to improve your sleep or to seriously take on any sleep issues, just as it isn't enough to sprinkle sleepy scents on to your pillow, breathe deeply for a few minutes and expect sleep to come. A sleep script is one part of a 360-degree approach that encompasses healthy sleep habits for your body and daily routine, and the suggestions you're giving yourself. Combine those and you will have a strategy you can run with.

By understanding the basic science of sleep and what needs to be going on in your body to keep your sleep–wake cycle running smoothly, you're also making your sleep script that much more effective. Professor Peter Whorwell's Manchester hospital department discovered that it is the only way to get results that last when treating patients with extreme and persistent IBS.

Suggestion appears to be so simple on the surface (as Coué put it, 'the simplest thing in the world', writing on another occasion, 'There are those who cannot imagine so simple a thing will produce such an effect! Because it is too easy to understand!'). But we've already seen how much it can control: our body chemicals, emotions, moods, personality, habits, reality, pain levels, confidence, health, mindset, behaviour, and our brain's priorities and neural pathways. And how it can be turbocharged and embedded for the long term when it is backed up by an understanding of what's supposed to be going on in a healthy body, and in a sleep–wake cycle that's firmly on track. With this appreciation of all these factors, now is the right time to introduce a sleep script, because you are armed with all this knowledge and can therefore understand how effective a sleep script can be on many different levels.

A stage set for sleep

Waters' sleep script is short compared to others I've come across subsequently, but it was effective for me and he explained that he wrote it to 'train the system to proper conditions of sleep', adding, 'An excellent time to train this suggestion into the mind is while resting comfortably in a chair before the evening meal. Either read it quietly aloud to yourself or have it read to you.'

You could either record yourself reading one of the scripts below, as I did, or you could record someone else reading it, if their voice sounds relaxing and velvet smooth. Professor Whorwell says that in his experience someone else's voice works best, so if you can find the right voice for your ears, so much the better. But with any script, the trick is to read it, or to have it read, at a slow, gentle pace, with lots of pauses, to slow you right down, to make you more receptive and give your brain time to absorb the messages being sent its way.

Ideally, you should try to listen to a script in the same place at the same time each day, as the associations wrapped up with a particular setting send a very clear signal to the brain, giving instant impact – the expectations carrying a weighty influence of their own. If you can choose a particular armchair, room or park bench, your brain will know what's about to happen and you'll feel more relaxed and in the zone, even before the script starts to roll.

That wasn't an option for me, although I did set a 5pm alarm on my phone to anchor the script to this part of the day, and I would try to listen to it then or soon after. A 6pm or 7pm reminder might suit your lifestyle better, but only you will know the most convenient early evening time slot for you.

I used to really enjoy this tranquil pause in the day. It was instantly soothing – a mindful moment. And hearing those positive sleep suggestions, murmured daily into my ears, was not only relaxing and reassuring, but I could also see the effect of the script gathering strength day by day. When heading off to bed, or in bed, however many hours later, I'd often think about Waters' script and the odd words or phrases that I could remember, which were surprisingly powerful for calming both my mind and body, and for reminding my brain what was expected of it. And given that the brain loves certainty, responds to instruction and works by predicting the future, the words in the script spelt out very clearly what that immediate future was going to be: Deep. Revitalising. Sleep.

Once the deed is done, you can carry on with your evening, reassured in the knowledge that when you do make the decision in your head that you're going to bed to go to sleep, or out loud to anyone who's around (for greater effect), your body and mind will start to automatically go into sleep-preparation mode. Both body and mind will calm down: shedding residual fight-or-flight symptoms left over from your day, relaxing into rest and digest, reducing brain chatter and stress chemicals, upping the sleepy hormone melatonin and GABA (as darkness descends), which shuts down your wide-awake system.

I don't listen to Waters' recording any more, as I tend to sleep well and wake rested, and I know what action to take in the moment if anything starts to slip. But I still have the recording in my phone's voice memos in case something ruffles my sleep and I need to reinforce my good sleep habits, as happened briefly at the beginning of the coronavirus pandemic, with all the uncertainty and lack of structure that came with that. And on the odd other occasion that I have listened to it since ironing out my sleep – for example, when illness disrupts my rest – it sounds like an old, reassuring friend that instantly makes me feel relaxed, supported and on top of my sleep–wake cycle and my old, exhausting anti-sleep habits.

Story time

Your brain likes 'can do' messages, so when it comes to any suggestion, it's best *not* to tell yourself *not* to do something, I was told by Dr Syed Shariq Hasan, who talked me into a state of restful alertness in Chapter 1. The brain likes *dos*, he explained, so give it plenty of those. To take back control, you could say, 'I *can* smoke, but I don't want to. I *can* eat this unhealthy snack, but I don't want to. I *can* go to bed/sleep at 2am, but I don't want to ...'

Dr Hasan's office, as I mentioned in Chapter 1, is filled to overflowing with thank-you cards from patients he has treated with clinical hypnosis for various disorders, including insomnia. Stacked ten deep, the cards thank him for giving people their lives back with messages such as, 'Thank you for reprogramming my brain and body.'

'We can use the past in a negative or a positive way,' he tells me, citing one patient who cried when she told him about an old boss who used to bully her. 'She was still letting those memories ruin her present.' And when Dr Hasan discovered this boss had in fact died 40 years ago, he said, 'Where is he now? You're letting him bully you from nowhere.' Likewise, we can acknowledge that our sleep pattern used to be bad, but it's going to get better. Our past doesn't have to control or dictate our present or our future. 'The whole story changes, if you change your perception,' says Dr Hasan. Just as our sleep patterns can change, if we alter our perceptions, expectations, self-talk and our physiology and behaviour in line with that, with the help of a sleep script.

Sleep scripts

Waters' sleep script worked very well for me with its repeated, sleep-inducing suggestions. No doubt it helped that it was so short, which made it possible for me always to fit it into my day, although a longer script would have given me more time to relax and to get into a more receptive, meditative state.

This is why I have included two additional bespoke sleep scripts. Written exclusively for this book by two leading experts, they're suitable if you're looking for something longer that can work with your timetable and is more the experience you want from a sleep script.

One of the sleep scripts below has been written by the highly qualified cognitive hypnotherapist and executive mind coach Kirsty Macdonald, and although significantly longer than Waters' script, it is still something that can easily fit into the busiest of days and be listened to even when you're on the move, as long as you can find some uninterrupted time alone.

Where Waters' script is instructive, in a very sparse and straight-forward way, Macdonald's script is much more soothing, melodic and hypnotic, giving you the space to become more self-aware, so that you can slow down and relax. This will get your cortisol levels down, while allowing the natural rhythms of the body to take over, with, as she suggests: 'Your body and mind working together for you.'

The second, longer, sleep script, provided by Dr Hasan, gives access to the expertise of the ground-breaking hospital department he works in, run by Professor Peter Whorwell, which uses clinical suggestion backed up by recorded scripts to treat a wide range of disorders, including pain, phobias and insomnia. It's a cutting-edge approach to medicine that statistically gets dramatic results and which, previous to this script, was only available to hospital patients and staff.

If you have the time, the longer, *c.*11-minute script will, of course, get your cortisol levels down even further and give you the physiological benefits that come with meditation, such as a calm central nervous system and a reversal of the damage caused by stress at a molecular level, as previously discussed. The extra time will help to put you into a deeper meditative state, receptive to the suggestions being given. All of this will help improve your sleep.

Either way, whichever script you choose will help you to re-write your sleep thought habits, and your sleep behaviour, as both have been written by experts who have specifically worked with the power of suggestion to improve health and sleep, making them a perfect support for this book and this sleep method. It's just a matter of what appeals to you. You're in safe hands.

Kirsty Macdonald's sleep script

Executive mind coach and cognitive hypnotherapist Kirsty Macdonald's sleep-inducing script was written specifically for this book. Macdonald believes that it takes Waters' script to another level, given how much more we know about cognitive therapy compared to 100 years ago. The wording and punctuation are both carefully chosen for maximum effect.

The slower pace, relaxed reflection and the deep breathing she encourages will, as we've learnt, naturally slow brainwaves down, the purpose being to make the mind receptive to the positive sleep suggestions that are embedded in the script.

Before listening to a recording of the script, Macdonald advises that you, 'Sit somewhere warm and comfortable where you will not be disturbed (switch off your devices!). Take five deep breaths deep into your abdomen, imagine your body becoming heavier and more relaxed and slowly read or listen to a recording of this':

The script

As you approach time for your body and mind to rest and sleep, you could just begin to become aware of whatever it is you might need to experience more of, or perhaps less of, in order for you to begin to relax more and more. Whether it might be something you do on the outside of you that helps you to let go more fully – possibly a warm bath, candles or soft music. Or perhaps it's those feelings and thoughts on the inside – simply seeing or imagining the words 'calm and relaxed' and noticing so much more of where those feelings might live in your body if they were to become more present now. Or quite possibly both, or something else entirely that could begin to come to you now. So you could just begin to more fully allow the possibility of your body doing exactly what it already knows how to do, as it slows down and relaxes more and more, in order for you to experience so much more of a restful night's sleep.

And whether you remember exactly what makes the difference, or perhaps forget to remember to pay attention at all, just means that as you begin to allow the wisdom of your body and mind to come through as it relaxes, you can be sure that sleep is the most natural thing in the world. And just like all the other natural things your body does each day, like breathing itself, it's really about just allowing it to happen rather than being in the doing of anything in particular ...

So if you were to *slow right down now* and imagine what it would be like to completely forget to do anything that might previously have gotten in the way of your just being able to sleep restfully now, you might even be curious to notice what it might be about this new way of being that could even be enjoyable in some way. Your body and mind working together for you. Forgetting to remember to pay attention to those old patterns because this is about a new way of letting go of the mind and relaxing the body. So it might only be the second or third time that you notice getting so much more of the sleep you want that you notice for the first time how much has changed. And then it's just a question of that 'calm and relaxed', or whatever else it is that you experience in these moments, becoming so much more of who you are now, just naturally. Your body resting, your mind relaxing. Your journey into sleep, in whatever way it occurs, increasingly becoming a gift to yourself.

Dr Syed Shariq Hasan's sleep script

Public health specialist and clinical hypnotherapist, Dr Syed Shariq Hasan, based at Manchester University NHS Foundation Trust (MFT), has also written a longer bespoke sleep script for *Teach Yourself to Sleep*, based on the format he uses to talk his patients into a state of restful alertness, a state of mind that's most receptive to suggestion and achieved only in deep relaxation and transcendental meditation.

Now, with Dr Hasan's script, you could either listen to this earlier in the evening, as I did with Waters', or if you really want to listen to this in bed (although ideally you want to keep this a tech-free zone, as much as possible), there are two alternative endings, as you'll see below.

The day-time/night-time script

Just take a deep breath and relax now. Breathe in and breathe out and keep on relaxing. Every breath that you take out, takes you deeper and deeper down into relaxation, and as you go deeper and deeper down into relaxation, you become more and more aware of yourself. You become aware of your breathing, you become aware of your bodily sensations, you become aware of everything happening within and around you. Your awareness of everything happening within and around you is becoming stronger and stronger with every breath you take out.

As you go into a deeper and deeper state of relaxation, you can feel a bit of tension in your body that might interfere with the process of relaxation.

[Long pause]

In order to get rid of all this tension from your body, I would now request your subconscious mind to mentally scan your body for areas of tension, and make note of how your body feels.

Notice how your body feels right now. Where in your body is today's tension stored?

Focus your attention on that part of the body that feels most tense. Start to focus on that area of tension.

You will now gradually focus on releasing all the tension in your body that you have found and start to quieten your mind.

So breathe in slowly and deeply, and then let the tension go as you breathe out with a sigh.

[Long pause]

You can feel yourself releasing all the tension from your body.

Every time you breathe out, you exhale all the tension from your body.

Now notice where your body feels most relaxed and let the feeling of relaxation grow with each breath that you're taking, spreading further and further the feeling of relaxation.

What a wonderful feeling of relaxation. What a comfortable feeling.

You're feeling so relaxed and you're feeling so comfortable.

Once the mind is calm and peaceful, you'll easily drift into a pleasant, restful sleep.

You might have thoughts about things you did today. About things you need to do tomorrow. Perhaps you are worried about something or someone. Now is the time to clear your mind for sleep, so tomorrow you will be refreshed and strong and can handle your duties and roles efficiently. Now take a few moments to do the thinking you need to do before you go to sleep. Anything you need or want to think about before you go to sleep. For the next few moments do any worrying or thinking you decide to do. Just take a few moments and do all the worrying or thinking you decide to do.

[Long pause]

As you've done all the thinking and worrying, now is the time to clear your mind for sleep. There's nothing else you need to do at this moment. Nothing you need to be thinking about except calm, relaxed thoughts. Now feel your attention drifting as you become sleepy and calm.

[Long pause]

You can feel the waves of relaxation flowing down your body.

Imagine a wave of relaxation starting from the top of your head. It relaxes the muscles in your scalp. It then goes down into your face, relaxing the muscles in your face, passing into your neck, relaxing all the muscles in your neck, going into your shoulders, relaxing all the muscles in your shoulders. And from your shoulders it goes into your upper arms, relaxing the muscles in your upper arms, passing your elbow joints into your forearms, relaxing the muscles in your forearms, passing through your wrists into your hands, relaxing each and every muscle in your hands and reaching your fingertips. What a wonderful feeling of relaxation, as the wave of relaxation flows all the way down from the top of your head, through your shoulders and arms into your fingertips, relaxing and comforting each and every part of your upper limb, head and neck.

And now this wave of relaxation flows down into your back, relaxing the muscles in your back, it goes into your chest, relaxing the muscles in your chest. Your lungs are expanding and your breathing becomes more and more comfortable and you feel more and more relaxed all over your chest. It goes down into your abdomen, relaxing the muscles in your abdomen, completely relaxed. And from your abdomen it goes into your bottom, relaxing the muscles in your bottom, passing through your thighs, relaxing the muscles in your thighs, passing through your knee joints into your legs, relaxing each and every muscle in your leg, passing through your calf muscles, your ankle joints and into your feet, relaxing each and every muscle in your feet and reaching the tips of your toes. What a wonderful feeling of relaxation. As a wave of relaxation goes all the way down from the top of your head to the bottom of your spine, your fingertips and the tips of your toes. Every muscle in your body is now relaxing into this lovely state. What a wonderful feeling of relaxation. What a comfortable feeling.

From now on each night, night after night, as
you prepare to go to bed, a feeling of calmness and
preparedness for sleep will emerge and you'll be able
to feel completely relaxed and at ease, feeling calm
and tranquil. Knowing that every day is another day
complete and knowing that tomorrow will be another
opportunity to experience new challenges. So from
now on, as you move forward from this point, as you
prepare to go to sleep, every night will be calm, more
and more calm, each and every night. You'll
be at ease, more and more at ease. Your mind and
your body will be relaxed. Released from any stress
and tension and totally rested. You'll be able to sleep
with tranquillity, confidence, deeply and securely
free and at peace, the best sleep you ever had. Sleep
as you did as a small child, as a baby, undisturbed,
settled sleep, as you are totally immersed in deep
relaxing sleep. Calmly and deeply relaxed. You're able
to use all the noises of the world to deeply soothe
your sleep, totally at peace.

So from now on, you'll sleep so soundly. You'll
allow your imagination and your creativity to offer
deep and undisturbed calmness, a restful calmness,
a deep and restful calmness, completely rested. You'll
be able to sleep soundly, knowing in the back of your
mind that day by day you are beginning to live more
fully and more deeply. As time goes on, you will live
with more and more wisdom and confidence, and
you will let yourself sleep the way a baby does, as
the baby feels peaceful and very secure. You'll sleep
wonderfully easily. Very restfully, with a calmness and
depth just right for you.

After a peaceful night's sleep you will wake up at the right time to start your day. As you wake in the morning, you'll wake from a deep, restful, relaxing, calm sleep, feel fully satisfied from your deep, restorative sleep. You'll feel refreshed, very well and very calm. And when you wake up in the morning, you'll be completely refreshed and totally energised and invigorated to take on the challenges of the day, the week and the life ahead of you.

So from now on you'll begin your day feeling increasingly energised and excited about the new opportunities the day has to offer. This increasing feeling of energy will begin as soon as you wake up, feeling energised, enthused and inspired, totally inspired, immersed in joy, so energetic, full of this energising positivity, with the readiness to experience the new opportunities that are waiting for you to experience as you clamber readied from your restful bed, into the waiting day. Because of this you'll wake up with an overwhelming eagerness to get up from your bed, to clamber into the new awaiting world. You may want to experience the day as soon as it begins and on those days, you'll wake easily feeling refreshed and alert, whilst on other days, you'll sleep soundly and peacefully until you need to wake, rise and enter the day.

Every day, day by day, you'll wake with more and more energy, feeling able and enthusiastic to be fully involved in the day. You'll feel so vibrant and energised, alert, calm, totally focused, very well organised. You'll feel in control and refreshed and yet relaxed, with bags and bags of energy, a total feeling of contentment, more and more happy. Happier and happier. More and more satisfaction and well-being with every waking moment. And as your day evolves, you'll maintain this inner feeling of contentment and satisfaction, happiness, calm soothing happiness, feeling more and more alert, calm and increasingly satisfied, with a sense of success, vibrancy and creativity, a feeling of resilience and energised calmness. Feeling a calm, energised vibrant energy within your body, and as you surface from your invigorating, refreshing sleep, as you wake in the morning, you'll feel so good, you'll feel so nice and so comfortable, you'll wake so refreshed. You will wake so energised and run through the plan of the day ahead, ready and prepared to enjoy the new day ahead of you.

So every day, you'll feel more alert, more refreshed, more calm, complete focus, strong and healthy, because you will have slept soundly, deeply, securely and at peace, knowing that each day and every day life is continuing, just as life continues, you'll find more and more joy in your life and just as surely as time goes on, you'll continue to grow and grow in your contentment and your calmness and your understanding of what you need to do, to immerse yourself in effective rest patterns. Just as you will grow more and more aware of how nature finds balance in the world, you'll become more and more aware of how to get balance in your own world, balance in your work time, your leisure time, your rest time, so that you fully experience all aspects of life.

This will happen just as I say it will happen,

because from now on you will establish good night-time routines. When you prepare for sleep, you will feel ready to sleep because you will go to bed with a feeling of calmness and preparedness for sleep and you'll be able to feel completely relaxed and at ease, feeling calmly relaxed, calm, knowing that every day is another day complete. Starting now, as you go to bed, you will retire ready to have a deep sleep and you will enjoy the deep sleep, knowing you will sleep like a baby, so peacefully and so calmly. You'll use simple breathing techniques to maintain your calmness and know that your skills at self-administrative sleep will support you. You'll feel calm throughout your life. Every night you'll be calm and tranquil. Every night at ease, your mind and your body will be calm, tranquil and relaxed. You'll be able to sleep calmly, soundly, securely and at peace. You'll be able to sleep as you did as a baby. So calm. So untroubled. So relaxed. So completely at peace.

Day-time ending

You are feeling so relaxed and comfortable. Getting rid of all the stress and tension from your mind has made you feel so refreshed and energised that you look forward to enjoying the rest of the day and cherish each and every moment of your life.

Take all the time you need to relax now and then gradually begin to bring yourself back just whenever you feel ready to do so.

So take a deep breath now and slowly open up your eyes.

Feeling refreshed and energised for the rest of the day.

Night-time ending

As you're feeling so relaxed right now, you are going deeper and deeper down into relaxation, into a deep, restful pleasant sleep.

And you're doing it right now. You're now sleeping like a baby. It's calm, it's peaceful, it's tranquil, going into a deeper and deeper state of sleep right now, going deeper and deeper down into a deeper state of relaxation. Feeling so calm and so tranquil. Going into a deeper state of sleep right now. Feeling so calm and so tranquil, you're sleeping like a baby, going deeper and deeper down into relaxation, sleeping like a baby right now, deeper and deeper state of relaxation, so just let go and relax now.

Repetition is key, as it is with any effective suggestion, or new habit, as we've seen throughout this book, be that self-motivating self-talk, a sleep-biology suggestion, or creating a new sleep-routine habit to sideline an old unwanted one. Although I no longer listen to Waters' script daily, because this habit/need naturally tailed off, at some point, the new sleep pattern I was working on, along with the thought and behavioural changes that back it up, have all stuck. As Waters wrote, which I quoted in Chapter 4, 'The amount of impression which we can obtain by one direct suggestion is limited, while the amount we can build up by repetition is unlimited.'

If you would like to access free audio downloads of the above scripts, read by Kate Mikhail, Kirsty Macdonald and Dr Syed Shariq Hasan, please visit katemikhail.com.

4 top tips

1. Set a daily sleep-script reminder, for some time before your evening meal.
2. Listen to a sleep script somewhere quiet or alone.
3. Use a sleep script as a calming pause in your day and as a suggestive sleep-habit cue.
4. Think back to your sleep script as you head to bed.

Chapter 10

From the Outside In

And then there's your sleep-habit context and personal
reward zone, plus those top-of-the-list sleep-habit cues.

Coué and Waters dealt with insomnia on a deep, internal level, using
suggestion to tap into our autopilot selves – the 'madman at home'
that is an out-of-control imagination and our subconscious – to shift
patterns of thought and behaviour in order to get real, physical results.
And although there's no doubt that the lack of screens 100 years ago,
with their blue-white lights, meant those night-and-day signals being
fired at our brains were more in line with the rising and setting of the
sun, there have always been external reasons why people have not been
able to sleep easily. These need to be considered, too.

As with repeated suggestions practised by Coué and Waters, our
environmental cues and repeated actions also create new habits, so
this is about setting up and focusing on the sleep cues around you
that you want your brain to absorb, while removing others that are
undermining your sleep.

The bigger the nest, the better

OK, so, you're lying in bed. Your sleep drive is high. GABA and sleepy melatonin levels are up there, stress chemicals are low, brainwaves are slowing down and your body clocks are ticking together, all holding hands, but just as you're about to go to sleep, you become aware of that bump in the mattress, and snap to. No matter where you roll you can't get comfortable, someone else's hot breath is in your face, your pillow is giving you a crick in the neck, you stretch and hit a limb from the other side of the bed, a motorbike roars by ... and sleep is snatched away from you. Just. Like. That.

We might be able to tweak our moods, emotions, personality, body chemicals, physiology, pain levels, health, reality, thought and behaviour habits, imagination, cognitive function, outlook, our brain's priorities, and our sleep ... (and breathe) ... by using suggestion in its various guises. But we also need to recognise that 25 per cent of sleep problems can be blamed on partner disturbance, according to the Sleep Council's Great British Bedtime Reports; a further 20 per cent on noise, and 13 per cent on an uncomfortable bed, so practical and luxury add-ons that double as positive sleep-habit cues can really help.

Remember when you were a child you probably had a single bed about 90cm (3ft) wide? How much space do you have now, given that you're an adult and that much bigger? The size and comfort of your bed is crucial. And bigger is definitely better, particularly if you're sharing your bed with someone else. Your bed/mattress also needs to tick that habit-reward box, so that going to bed is something your brain looks forward to, and your new sleep habits have that fifth building block to stick to: dopamine hit guaranteed, oxytocin as well. Deliciously comfortable. Your time to relax. Without being disturbed.

This is a purchase that can't be rushed. Ideally, you want to head to some of the biggest bed shops you can find, selling the kind of mattress that you're looking for (sprung, latex, memory foam, futon, smart bed, gel, air, adjustable, organic – whatever suits you best) and give yourself hours of time to bed-surf until you find one that's perfect for you (and your budget) and you can feel your body sighing with relief, wishing it was time for sleep. Measure away, to be sure of the space you're getting. A UK double bed (not the small double) is 135 ′ 190cm (the traditional 4ft 6in-wide double bed). Next is the kingsize at 150 ′ 200cm (or 5ft – called a queensize in the US), then there's the super-kingsize at 190 ′ 200cm (6ft – in the US the super-king is 6.33ft). Although there are beds wider than this, of course, you can see that getting the 90cm (3ft) you had as a child is not a given when you're sharing.

Bed-buying tips

One tip is to try lying on your side on the floor before you head off to the store. Can you feel how uncomfortable that is? All those curves and bones that are *not* sinking into the floor? When you lie on your side on your mattress, you should sink in all the way along your body so that your spine looks straight, side-on, while you are absorbed and supported. For that you need something that's soft and forgiving on the top layer but firmer at its core.

The lighter you are, the softer the mattress you need, otherwise you'll barely make an impression on it. The heavier you are, the firmer the mattress to make sure you get the support you need. Split mattresses work well for couples, for this reason, so that both sides sleep soundly, the lighter side doesn't roll in to the dip made by the heavier side and neither side wakes up with backache from a night on a mattress that's too hard or too soft for their body weight. Some brands will even let you try out a mattress for comfort at home, offering you your money back if you don't sleep well on it. I used to have a mattress that was far too hard and unforgiving for me, leaving me lying on the surface rather than sinking in and supported. Now I have a natural latex one, although I'm tempted to make the surface that much more cushioned with a woollen, heat-diffusing topper. Toppers are, of course, an effective and less pricey way to turn a so-so mattress into a really comfortable one and offset those pressure points. But any which way, total comfort needs to be assured.

Make a habit of it

Routine. Cues. Reward. Stand-ins. Repeat. Habit context – in other words, your bedroom – is the strongest of cues, as discussed in Chapter 4, so creating a bedroom that's a haven-cum-reward zone is critical to overturning old sleep habits, as well as setting off your happy neuro-transmitters and a cascade of positive sleep associations for your new sleep habits to grab on to.

This involves making your bedroom as inviting and sleep-friendly as possible: comfortable bed, clean, dust-free, lovely, natural-fibre bedding (more effective for staying cool), clutter-free, nice smelling with no work or distractions that are going to engage you mentally and pull you out of that sleep countdown at night. As we saw on page 89 I found overhauling my bedroom to be an extremely satisfying, pro-active part of tackling my chronic insomnia once I'd learnt about how thought and behaviour habits are made in the brain and how they can be derailed and new habits built.

There are many things that you can add to make a bedroom your ideal space. Electronic air purifiers are said to spruce up air quality, reducing unwanted odours, allergens and gases, the idea being that they can help those with dust-mite allergies or hay fever by cleaning the air and making the sleeper less congested, and therefore more able to sleep soundly, although reviews are mixed.

Bedroom plants are good to have around, given that they absorb carbon dioxide and release oxygen, which upgrades the air quality. NASA has given the top air-purifying-plant award to the chrysanthe-mum, so you might want a bunch of flowers from this outdoor plant to add colour to your room, although the peace lily, snake plant, bamboo palm, spider plant and others also do a good job of cleaning air. Bedrooms also need to be cool – ideally 17°C (62.6°F), according to latest research, to give you the best chance of not upsetting your body clocks by getting too cold or overheating and waking in the night.

Essential oils are also affordable and effective sleep-habit cues that bring more than a nice scent to a bedroom. Whether inhaled or absorbed through the skin (in baths, or as the new generation of perfumes with a job to do), they've been shown time and again to relieve stress and anxiety, and to improve sleep. Put some on your bedding, in a burner or a diffuser before you go to bed, or use a smart diffuser that will pump out different smells at different times of the day, and you can fill your room with delicious, calming, soporific smells – lavender, chamomile, sweet orange, rose, ylang ylang and cedarwood, are considered some of the best for reducing anxiety and inducing relaxation and sleep (with lavender at the top of the list). Plus, stepping into an exquisite olfactory heaven will help set off your sensory reward system.

All afloat

Picture-perfect bedrooms piled high with pillows are *not* what your body's looking for. I always sling those extra pillows to one side when I'm staying anywhere and hope that there's a pillow in there that's not going to be too solid, high or uncomfortable. One pillow I had on a trip to the States was unbelievable: I could feel myself floating off into sleep faster than usual, my head melting into a fluffy cloud, while supported at the same time (soft on the outside, firm at the core). It set me off on a quest to find something similar in the UK, taking into account the arguments about flame retardants, off-gassing and chemicals in bedding (and mattresses) and the effect this can have on our health. Laws are different in this respect the world over and are changing all the time.

Awareness of off-gassing (also called out-gassing) is big in the United States. This is when household products release potentially harmful chemicals and particles into the air: volatile organic compounds (VOCs – that smell you get with new carpet, bedding or a sofa, for example), which is why so many products are advertised as being free from harmful chemicals, with limited or no off-gassing. Wool is naturally fire-resistant, so this is often used as the upper layer/

covering in pillows and mattresses (and furnishings) that are free of flame-retardants, chemicals and off-gassing.

For snorers, new pillows every six months or anti-allergy pillows (using natural latex foam) are recommended to cut down on dust mites in the bedroom, which will ease congestion and help to reduce snoring, making sleep that much more restorative. And for really comfortable sleep, all most people need is a slim pillow that fills the gap between your head and the mattress, to support your head and keep your spine straight.

If you're a side sleeper (rather than a front or back sleeper), you'll need a slightly higher pillow to fill the gap and keep your spine and neck in line. If you're someone who changes position throughout the night, a medium-height pillow is your best option. With some mattresses you won't even need this, if your body sinks in far enough that there is no gap. As with mattresses, however, you need to find the right pillow for your sleep position and sense of comfort. Pillows that leave you pummelling or fidgeting to get comfortable will make you more aware and 'on' than you want to be before sleep, and the wrong pillow can leave you overheating, or with neck ache that can interrupt your sleep.

To have and to hold

An abrupt snort. Up close. Rhythmic, irritating snoring. Loud, heavy breaths. The odd snuffle or snore here and there, and the tension-filled silences in between while you wait, slightly stressed (and possibly annoyed) and alert for the next snort, snore or snuffle from the other side. All of these can really set off that insomnia panic, anxiety and/or mounting rage that kisses sleep goodbye.

Partners are often blamed for ruining sleep, which, presumably, is why surveys show an increasing number of people are choosing to sleep apart (estimated at 25-plus per cent) and many more would like to, even if they don't admit this to the outside world (or even to their partner), for fear of being judged or it being assumed that their relationship is on the rocks. There are two camps on this. On the one side, the 'You take the bed. I'll take the sofa bed/spare bedroom' sleep-divorce idea is seen as a sensible solution that safeguards sleep *and* improves the relationship by making both parties more rested and nocturnal visits more fun/appealing, but on the other it's damned as a marriage breaker that strips a relationship of intimacy. Part-time sleep divorces are thought to be more common than we realise; say, if one person comes home late, having been out on the town (so takes the sofa), either one is ill, or has a different work or sleep–wake schedule, or a child or two has crawled into the marital bed.

It's obviously a case of what works for you and yours. But the main thing with sharing a bed is that both sleepers' patterns and require-ments need to be equally prioritised. If one wants to read and the other wants to go straight to sleep, bedtimes might need to be staggered, for example. And if you're fighting over the duvet in the middle of the night, individual duvets (and electric blankets) can deal with this. Or you could opt for a vast duvet that swamps your mattress, providing plenty of cover for two.

Eye shades (silk lets your eyes 'breathe', instead of getting hot and puffy, although there are lots of eye-shade options on the market) and earplugs are, of course, cheap and simple light-and-sound barriers if you don't want to move to another room (or don't have the luxury of that choice).

Earplugs don't stop you actually hearing, but they can muffle the noise enough for you to fall asleep. Foam, wax, silicone, multi-use, whichever earplug you go for it's worth experimenting and finding the right size for your ear canal, so that they are really comfortable. White noise/sleep machines and other noise-masking systems are put forward as another way to counteract noise pollution from inside and outside the bedroom, and can come with a whole range of ambient and soothing sounds, from standard white noise (gentle static) and fan sounds to natural ones, which are said to envelop and neutralise the one keeping you awake.

I've never tried one, as I haven't felt the need enough, plus a 2020 systematic review of how effective white noise machines are for helping with sleep, carried out by a team at the University of Pennsylvania School of Medicine, concluded that the evidence in their favour is very low. The sound of water rushing over a weir outside a place I regularly visit in France, however, always seems to soothe me into a particularly deep sleep.

No laughing matter

Snore at night, and the chances are you will be wiped out during the day. The two are linked. And the more intense the snoring, the worse your daytime sleepiness.

Snoring – which is the sound of a vibrating tongue, throat and airways – affects about 90 million American adults, according to the National Sleep Foundation, and 45 per cent of British adults. It is very common in those over the age of 40, but it is not something we should mask or ignore in the long term, or laugh at or dismiss as irritating (although irritating it can be), without trying to do something about it.

The reality is, scientists have discovered that habitual snoring and daytime sleepiness and fatigue go hand in hand – snoring being a sign that your breathing is obstructed, with oxygen having to fight its way through those vibrating muscles, soft tissues and tongue, which means that you're far from getting the best sleep possible. Sort out your snoring and your daytime energy levels will go up. Ignore the problem and not only will you be more exhausted during the day, but on-going snoring can damage the airways and lead to hypopnea, or obstructive sleep apnoea (see page 201), which is when you momentarily stop breathing and starve your body of oxygen.

Sometimes with snoring, all you have to do is roll the body into a different position – you can even buy T-shirts that have a pocket for a tennis ball on the back (or wear a T-shirt with a top pocket back to front), nice and uncomfortable, to keep the snorer on their side or front where their airways are not blocked. Other suggestions include raising the head end of your bed by several inches (by putting a block under the bed legs), using a pillow wedge, or a smart mattress or a bed that can tilt itself upwards at the head end, to keep the snorer more upright and their airways clear.

Throat muscles relax with age, which is why we're more likely to snore the older we get, but excess weight is also a major cause of snoring (although thin people can snore, too), as this fat leads to extra soft tissue in the throat and neck, which can put pressure on your throat muscles and airways. All of this means that losing a bit of weight can be an effective solution if you do snore (your doctor should be able to give advice on the best options for you).

Other causes include smoking, which can block airways by irritating the membranes in the nose and throat, and drinking alcohol, as this causes the neck and tongue muscles to relax even more than they usually do during sleep, and, as a result, get in the way of airflow; your tongue falls backwards, blocking your airflow, and everything else slightly collapses in on itself. This also happens when you take sedatives (tranquillisers, sleeping tablets or anti-histamines). Being congested when you're ill can also make you snore.

If, however, you've ticked all the boxes and tried every trick in the book – given up smoking, cut back on alcohol (especially before bed), lost some weight, toned up your muscles, and got your tennis ball in place – and nothing is working, it's then worth asking your doctor to check what other causes there might be. Allergies, adenoids, infections or nasal blockages are possibilities. Your doctor can then advise what can be done to sort out the problem to improve the quality of your sleep and your energy levels during the day. An underactive thyroid is also a treatable cause of snoring, so it's worth getting your thyroid checked.

You can also try changing your perception via auto-suggestion if you're being kept awake by a snorer. Taking a Coué 'No, that does not trouble me at all' approach, you can try to refocus your response so that instead of hearing the snoring as something that's intrusive or abrasive, you can choose to hear it as a rhythmic, melodic purr that you can roll with.

The wrong kind of silence – sleep apnoea

Snore. Silence. Gasp. This can be fatal. If the snoring coming from you or your partner involves long silences, followed by big gasps as air is urgently sucked in, this could be sleep apnoea, where you momentarily stop breathing due to relaxed throat muscles blocking the airway, before waking up (although you won't remember this) and sharply breathing in to force open the airways and to re-oxygenate the body. This is an urgent one for your doctor, as it will need to be monitored and action taken without delay.

Sleep apnoea – which means total obstruction (when no air can get through) – and hypopnoea (partial obstruction) is when a sleeper struggles between trying to breathe and choking. With hypopnoea airflow is reduced, but with obstructive sleep apnoea (OSA) it's stopped in its tracks and sleepers stop breathing altogether for anything from 10 seconds to minutes. Worldwide it's estimated that nearly a billion people have sleep apnoea, which can lead to chronic fatigue and long-term health risks. Not everyone is aware whether they suffer from this or not, but around half of those who snore loudly have sleep apnoea, according to the National Sleep Foundation.

It's not as if this is something that happens occasionally during the night, either. Sleepers with OSA can wake up 300–400 times in a night, and this broken sleep, which will drag you from a deep sleep to a shallow one in order to pull in some oxygen, will obviously leave you wrung out and sleep deficient, as well as it being potentially fatal.

If your doctor thinks you may be suffering from OSA, they will refer you to a sleep clinic where you'll either be given a polysomnography, with body sensors wired up to a computing system while you sleep, or you will be sent home with overnight equipment that you can work yourself to monitor your sleep. Mild apnoea is not generally seen as a problem, but in severe cases sleepers are given a continuous positive air pressure (CPAP) mask to sleep with. This keeps their airways open, using a constant flow of compressed air. Although a CPAP can take some getting used to, the positives are a huge improvement in your quality of life and energy levels, as well as taking away the risk of high blood pressure, having a stroke or heart attack or an irregular heartbeat that come with OSA.

From the inside out

You can cuddle a robot to help you sleep, wear high-tech pyjamas to regulate your body temperature, use sleep trackers and apps and weighted gravity blankets, or wear headbands to stimulate your brain, but there's no magic gadget that can serve up natural, refreshing sleep on a platter if your sleep pattern is in chaos and you're not dealing with the underlying biological, habitual or suggestion-based causes.

With the sleep-aid market set to be worth an estimated $101.9 billion, covering everything from sleeping pills to sleep apnoea monitors, bedding and gizmos, the human quest for first-rate sleep has become big business. And while some sleep tech can, of course, help you to relax, cool down and switch off from our hyper-connected, over-stimulating lifestyle, if you can afford it, this is only part of the battle.

One thing I have ended up investing in for the family are blue-light-blocking glasses. These boost melatonin levels by cutting out blue light that suppresses melatonin, and they have cut down arguments about screen time, or about the need to check phones last thing (although not completely).

Ironically, some sleep tech can be counter-productive. By obsessively checking our sleep data, doctors say we can end up stressing out about sleep problems that might not even exist. And this stress can then disrupt sleep that was fine in the first place, or just needed a little upgrade. Orthosomnia ('ortho' meaning correct, and 'somnia' meaning sleep) has now been recognised as a condition where sleepers become fixated on an unhealthy, tunnel-vision mission to achieve an almost competitive, 'perfect' sleep – by over-medicalising it to the point where they create an issue.

Instead of medicalising sleep in this way, especially if this adds to our stress or any sense of sleep failure, what we need to do is appreciate the simplicity of the sleep–wake cycle and recognise what, *specifically*, is sabotaging ours so that we can work with our minds, bodies, lifestyles and our environment to sort it out.

And by using some of the more practical sleep paraphernalia that's on offer – be that a mattress topper, anti-snore T-shirt, or blue-light blocking glasses, we can give ourselves a greater chance of having *quality* – not *perfect* – sleep that will recharge us, keep us healthy and set us up for each day.

4 top tips

1. Choose a mattress that keeps your spine straight (when lying on your side).
2. If you're light, choose a softer mattress; if you're heavier, a harder one.
3. Buy a pillow that just fills the gap between your head and bed.
4. Fill your bedroom with sensory rewards, to help cement your new sleep habits.

Chapter 11

The Protégé with a Crystal Ball

From science to you – birds that 'peek'
and 360-degree sleep.

'The idea of sleep creates sleep; the idea of sleeplessness creates sleeplessness,' wrote Coué. 'What is a person who sleeps well? It is a person who knows that when one is in the bed it is for sleep, and he sleeps.'

Coué's sudden death from emphysema and heart disease at the age of 69, having been a heavy smoker since the age of 13, saw the Coué empire disintegrate. His mortality evidently worked against him (especially given some of the wilder health claims linked to his name), as did the charlatans jumping on the Coué bandwagon, the in-fighting among some of his practitioners and the vigorous mud-slinging from those who had scoffed at, or been threatened by, his positive self-help message, church leaders who railed against the demystification of his cures and Freudians included.

If he had lived to a ripe old age, given his once global celebrity status, the impact he had on everyday lives and his sell-out tours, it seems more than likely that Coué might still be a household name today, much like Sigmund Freud and Franz Mesmer. Mesmer having left us with mesmerism, despite his controversial animal-magnetism theory that claimed we are filled with magnetic fluids that need to be balanced, which he first did with magnets, later using his hands and a metal wand.

As a press clipping summed up after Coué's first UK tour in 1922, 'M Coué has given us results. It is for science to discover and understand the mechanism by which these results are obtained, and, by that comprehension, to make them a permanent part of the heritage of humanity.' This is happening more and more. Particularly Waters' twist on the Coué Method, which is being taken up and developed by the world of science and medicine. Besides, Coué is still remembered in his native France, where a second international congress for the Coué Method was held in his home town of Nancy in 2017, and a monument to Coué stands in Nancy's Parc Sainte-Marie.

Despite Coué's abrupt exit from the world stage on 2 July 1926, Waters' practice, whose patients included members of London's high society, continued to expand long after the Coué boom years, thanks to his reputation, successes and the fashions of the day. As he explained: 'Psychological terms are so frequently bandied about in drawing-rooms and over the dinner table, that one is perhaps justified in saying that during the last decade the mind has taken the place of the stomach as a topical dinner-table subject. The Freudians and their various Nonconformist off-shoots have mainly been responsible for this popularising of the subject.'

Waters first ran a practice in Harley Street and later from a grandiose, eight-room mansion flat in Emperor's Gate, near Kensington Gardens in London, where he built up a clientele of wealthy, titled and artistic celebrities, as well as more modest families, too. He gave lectures on mind control for final-year students at the University of London, referred to himself as a practical psychologist, and wrote about being so inundated with work that he didn't need to promote himself, as word of mouth kept clients coming.

During the First World War, Waters worked as an ambulance

driver for the Red Cross, but he retreated from public life for a couple of years at the beginning of the Second World War, having been diagnosed with cancer, it's said, only to later return to work, apparently symptom-free and full of energy once again. Even when I knew him in his late seventies and late eighties, he was still visiting patients in their Knightsbridge mansions or receiving them at home, practising his biology-based suggestion method with his adored African grey parrot occasionally perched on the back of his chair. His positive outlook, good humour and love for life was as undiminished as ever – a small, framed picture of Coué positioned on his living-room mantelpiece.

My world of sleep

It's strange to think that if I hadn't decided to read Coué and Waters' books, which had been languishing in a corner for so many years, not only would I not have this window into their world and the work that they were both so passionate about, but I would also still be battling sleep and suffering all the negatives that go along with that.

It's no exaggeration to say that my life has been transformed by being able to sleep well, using the formula I've put together. I no longer stay awake half the night or wake up exhausted. My immune system is notably stronger, my emotions more even, my self-awareness and energy are up, while my stress levels are way down, and the burn-out days have stopped.

Being able to question emotions that I don't feel like having and swap them for others that make me feel better about where I am has also been an invaluable life skill that has rescued many a day, and made my sleep that much more effortless and deep. And I've got Coué and Waters to thank for this, as they inspired me to explore sleep and everything that impacts it from such a different perspective.

The thing to keep in mind in all of this is that sleep is not a standalone – something that's tacked on to the end of our day, as it is often presented. It is wrapped up with our mind–body loop, the stressors in our day, our thought and behaviour habits, the suggestions we give ourselves, our imagination and our version of reality. It is a product of our emotions and our body chemicals, the sleep–wake cues we live by, and whether or not we are lined up with the rising and setting of the sun, or blasting our circadian clocks into submission with an all-enveloping blue-white light.

On top of this, the march of science has given us so much more insight into ourselves, which we can use to understand and tune in to our sleep–wake life. How easily our cortisol levels can spike, for example. How self-talk can change us physically and cognitively. How the photoreceptors in our eyes react to night and day, or what sort of signals and data our brain relies on to choose our emotions – all of which affect our sleep.

The fact is we can all direct our brain one way or another, for starters by structuring our life around light and using suggestions that are well informed. We can nurture new habits, change our cellular make-up, bend reality in our favour and tame our imagination and, in the process, re-write our sleep–wake cycle.

I now reject what my imagination is offering if it's presenting me as an insomniac who is set to be awake most of the night, and I replace this with an image of myself fast asleep, reminding myself how well I sleep these days and knowing that this will have a real, immediate, physiological effect. I look at the sky all the time, conscious that this is re-setting my master body clock. I shoe-horn mini pauses into my day and try to step in as soon as possible to stop those sleep-blocking stress chemicals from rocketing, while cultivating the four happy hormones the best I can, and swapping negative emotions and perceptions for others that are, at the very least, more nuanced. I try to pay attention to the suggestions I give myself, to see if they are working with me or against me, and I regularly feed myself biology-based ones to support my sleep. I soak my nights in darkness, guard my melatonin, and visualise my brainwaves slowing down at night as I breathe deeply.

10, 9, 8 ...

Once you see sleep as something that's woven into your day, the result of a chemical sleep drive that slowly gathers momentum the longer you're awake, and your body's natural 24-hour sleep–wake rhythms (and circadian clocks), it soon becomes second nature to set up the right sleep-habit cues for this. I support those daily, sleep-inducing chain reactions with a sleep-enhancing schedule that's rooted in the biology and science of sleep and self-talk, and which starts the moment you wake up. Here's my schedule to count you down to sleep:

Sleep groove – day

10 Try to resist reaching for your computer or phone in the middle of the night if you can't sleep, as this is a sleep-sabotaging message that you don't want to give to your brain. The blue light will suppress your melatonin levels, the content will arouse your mind, and your desired sleep habit or pattern will be broken. Breathe deeply. Remember there's a fine line between resting and being asleep – and, besides, your sleep-inducing neurons have the upper hand, so, if left alone, your brainwaves will slow down and your flip-flop switch will take over once again. (In contrast, it's best to avoid dawdling in bed come morning, letting your mind wander. Your brain will again get the wrong idea: that it's OK to lie in bed, wide awake, letting your mind whirl or meander when it's light outside, or again last thing at night, when you're trying to go to sleep, when it's not.)

9 Let daylight flood in when you do wake (at the right time) in the morning. And open your eyes for your photoreceptors to take this in. Your master circadian clock needs to be shown that it's morning out there. It's time for melatonin to fully retreat, cortisol to step up, and the body's sleep-drive stopwatch to start running. Your bedtime routine starts here.

8 Structure your day using light. Anchor your morning in as much daylight as possible and sky-watch and light-grab throughout your day, all the time aware that this is syncing your body with the Earth's rotation and the rising and setting of the sun, and keeping your circadian clocks and your sleep routine on track.

7 Structure your day using food. Regular meals that we pause to register align our peripheral body clocks with our master dark–light body clock and the 24-hour clock outside, which will – when all synced – keep our sleep–wake cycle running smoothly. Sleep-friendly recipes and tryptophan-laden foods, including late-night snacks (no less than 30 minutes before bed), ensure the gut–brain–sleep loop functions at its best, and that the body is prepped for sleep at night.

6 Embrace routine. Sleep habits (any habits) need routine. Routine. Cues. Reward. Stand-ins. Repeat (see Chapter 4). This keeps your master circadian clock and molecular clocks in line with each other and with the 24-hour clock outside, and it makes it clear what's expected of them and when. Our clocks anticipate the sleep–wake cycle and the body chemicals and circadian rhythms that are needed at specific times of the day and night. And if you can stick to the same bedtime and wake-up time as much as possible, seven days a week, so much the better. This is the ideal. Your body *loves* routine.

5 Keep control of your cortisol levels, using stress busters, emotion swaps, self-talk and everything else we've learnt so that this stress hormone doesn't run riot and later disrupt your sleep. And be proactive about setting off the four happy hormones: dopamine (rewards), serotonin (mood lifters), endorphins (exercise and laughter) and oxytocin (sensuality).

Sleep groove – night

4 Read a sleep-inducing script early evening and let this self-talk/auto-suggestion/self-hypnosis/sleep-habit cue do its job – helping to rewire your habitual thoughts and automatic behaviour – while you carry on with your pre-sleep evening. And set a reminder, so that you don't forget this valuable pause in your day.

3 Structure your night using light. Create a dusk zone by dimming the lights, switching to red-spectrum lights or using candles as the night wears on, lining up your circadian clocks with the solar clock outside. Use blue-light filters for phones and computers and/or blue-light-blocking glasses. Take a pre-bed screen break. Enjoy an armchair off-load, if needed, in a dimly lit room. And make sure your bedroom is as dark as a pitch-black night sky.

2 Activate the clinical hypnotist within. Reinforce all the above as you go along with sleep-friendly suggestions, and in bed, if you need to, with a biological body scan and sleep-biology self-talk. Slow your breathing, breathe deep and think gently, in no particular order (or just be vaguely aware of the following): *I'm tired and ready for sleep and my sleep pressure is high. My body clocks are prepared for sleep, melatonin is gathering strength, GABA is shutting down my awake state* (then trigger an upsurge in both by staring into your pitch-dark bedroom). *My action chemicals, such as cortisol, have headed off for the night, my vagus nerve is carrying 'time for sleep' signals between my gut, body and brain. The more I breathe deeply, relax and react to the darkness, the calmer my central nervous system becomes, the greater my state of rest and digest and the slower and less intense my brainwaves, as they move from beta, to alpha and theta – making sleep inevitable. All of which will tip the balance, so that the flip-flop switch does its thing, and my brainwaves shift to delta.*

1 Tell yourself, 'I am going to sleep much better tonight' and later, 'I will be asleep soon', 'I am going to sleep now', or a similar mantra, knowing the power of suggestion and sleep-thought-habit cues that can change us physiologically and behaviourally. And repeat.

With this sleep-enhancing schedule I've put together, our sleeping life and our waking life are treated as one – with a 'sleep 360-degree' routine that works with the science and biology of sleep, acknowledging that the structure, hormones, behaviour, self-talk and biological rhythms of our days lead into our nights, and are all intertwined in a wake–sleep loop, which goes round again. And again.

United we doze

Some birds 'peek' while sleeping to keep a watchful eye on potential threats and predators. One eye opening, every now and then, or more often and for longer, depending on the threat. Marine mammals can swim and surface for air, alert to danger and obstacles, but with one half of their brain enjoying the electrical signals of slow-wave sleep. Transparent zebra fish reveal the 'pruning' of synapses and tidying up that goes on in the brain during sleep. And honey bees have stronger memories come morning if they're presented with an odour cue from their day while sleeping. It seems that most species in the animal kingdom sleep at some level, when they become less active and responsive, and this helps them to conserve energy and repair their central nervous system. It wasn't that long ago, however, when only birds and mammals were thought to sleep. This was before two ground-breaking, petri-dish-tapping lab experiments were carried out where flies dropped down with exhaustion, as if dead, after being deliberately kept awake.

Today, birds, mammals, rodents, fish, flies and scorpions are all being scrutinised for clues by scientists to see how they sleep and what this can tell us about human sleep, too.

Unihemispheric sleep, for example, is where one half of the brain slows down and sleeps while the other half stays awake, which is how birds are able to peek and dolphins and whales can keep going for days without total shutdown. Humans might not have this option at their disposal, but we can experience the 'first-night effect' when sleeping somewhere new, where one brain hemisphere remains more active than the other – ever vigilant until we feel safe. Sounds are picked up by the right ear during the light sleep phases and then transmitted to the more-awake left hemisphere – the side of the brain that's responsible for logic, analyses, thought and reasoning.

Sleep research is fascinating and ongoing. And whether it's our human need for seven hours plus, or the four hours that giraffes and elephants generally go for, or the fact that birds dream, too, and are thought to be able to sleep on the wing, or the ability of fur seals to swim on their side using one flipper while the other one rests – we clearly all need to sleep in order to reboot and function at our best.

The sleep–wake cycle is as natural as night follows day. If we can work *with* this 24-hour rhythm, then all is well inside. But if we ignore the way our body works and what it needs to sleep soundly at night, then we're setting ourselves up for troubled sleep and all the problems that go with that. Bad sleep habits can creep up on us, as we've seen, gathering strength the longer we let them run the show. But by understanding the biology and science of sleep and how easily habits can be created, you now have what it takes to send your mind, and therefore your body, the suggestions and habit cues you need to achieve deep, natural sleep tonight and for always.

Bibliography

Introduction: Why Bother Sleeping (Much) – and Where to Begin

Abad V. C. and Guilleminault C., 'Diagnosis and treatment of sleep disorders: a brief review for clinicians', *Dialogues Clin. Neurosci.* (2003); 5(4): 371–88.

Adams R. J. et al., 'Sleep health of Australian adults in 2016: results of the 2016 Sleep Health Foundation national survey', *Sleep Health* (2017); 3(1): 35–42.

Cappuccio F. P. et al., 'Quantity and quality of sleep and incidence of Type 2 diabetes: a systematic review and meta-analysis', *Diabetes Care* (2010); 33: 414–20.

Coué É., *Self Mastery by Conscious Autosuggestion*, the Lorraine Society of Applied Psychology (1921).

Coué, É., *How to Practice Suggestion and Autosuggestion*, American Library Service (1923).

Coué É. and Orton J. L., *Conscious Autosuggestion*, D. Appleton and Co (1924).

Coué É., 'Every day, in every respect …', *Self Mastery by Conscious Autosuggestion*, the Lorraine Society of Applied Psychology (1921), p20.

Coué É., 'What you need is some auto-suggestion': Orton, J. Louis: *Émile Coué – The Man and His Work* (1935), p74.

Coué É., 'I am not a healer ... I am not a magic maker ...': Coué, E: *How to Practice Suggestion and Autosuggestion* (1923), p108.

Coué É., 'Lord Curzon continues to sleep like a babe,' Orton, J. Louis: *Émile Coué – The Man and His Work* (1935), Chapter 13, p168.

'Recommended amount of seep for a healthy adult: a joint consensus statement of the American Academy of Sleep Medicine and Sleep Research Society', Consensus Conference Panel, *Sleep* (2015); 38(6)1: 843–844.

Eugene A. R. and Masiak J., 'The neuroprotective aspects of sleep', *Medtube Sci.* (2015); 3: 35–40.

Graci G. M. and Hardie J. C., 'Evidenced-based hypnotherapy for the management of sleep disorders', *International Journal of Clinical and Experimental Hypnosis* (2007); 55(3): 288–302.

Hafner M. et al.,'Why sleep matters – the economic costs of insufficient sleep: a cross-country comparative analysis', Santa Monica, CA: RAND Corporation (2016): https://www.rand.org/pubs/research_reports/RR1791.html.

Hobson J. A., 'Sleep is of the brain, by the brain and for the brain', *Nature* (2005); 437(7063): 1254–56.

Lancee J. et al., 'When thinking impairs sleep: trait, daytime and nighttime repetitive thinking in insomnia', *Behavioral Sleep Medicine* (2017); 15(1): 53–69.

Liu Y. et al., 'Relationships between housing and food insecurity, frequent mental distress, and insufficient sleep among adults in 12 US states, 2009', *Preventing Chronic Disease* (2014); 11: E37.

Marco H. et al., 'Why sleep matters – the economic costs of insufficient sleep: a cross-country comparative analysis', Santa Monica, CA: RAND Corporation (2016).

Nunn C. L. et al., 'Shining evolutionary light on human sleep and sleep disorders', *Evolution, Medicine, and Public Health* (2016); 1: 227–43.

Kohen D. P. and Olness K., *Hypnosis and Hypnotherapy with Children*, Fourth Edition, Routledge (2011).

Royal Society for Public Health. Vision, Voice and Practice: 'Waking up to the benefits of sleep', University of Oxford.

Schutte-Rodin S. et al., 'Clinical guideline for the evaluation and management of chronic insomnia in adults', *Journal of Clinical Sleep Medicine*: JCSM: Official Publication of the American Academy of Sleep Medicine (2008); 4(5): 487–504.

Schwartz J. R. and Roth T. 'Neurophysiology of sleep and wakefulness: basic science and clinical implications', *Current Neuropharmacology* (2008); 6(4): 367–78.

Schwegler K., Götzmann L. and Buddeberg C., 'Psychosocial and psychosomatic aspects of insomnia', Division of Psychosocial Medicine, University Hospital Zurich, *Arch. Neurol. Psychiatr.* (2003); 154: 310–15.

Shrivastava D. et al., 'How to interpret the results of a sleep study', *J. Community Hosp. Intern. Med. Perspect.* (2014); 4(5): 24983.

The Sleep Council, 'The Great British Bedtime Report', 2013 and 2017: www.sleepcouncil.org.uk.

Speirs R., great niece of Richard Waters: interviews with the author, February and March 2017.

Stranges S. et al., 'Sleep problems: an emerging global epidemic?', findings from the INDEPTH WHO-SAGE study among more than 40,000 older adults from 8 countries across Africa and Asia, *Sleep* (2012); 35(8): 1173–81.

The National Sleep Foundation: 'Sleep in America® Poll. Communications Technology in the Bedroom' (2011).

The National Sleep Foundation, 'Sleep Health Index®. Quarterly Report – Q4 2016'.

Thomas C. and Baker C. I., 'Teaching an adult brain new tricks: a critical review of evidence for training-dependent structural plasticity in humans', *NeuroImage, Elsevier Science B.V.*, Amsterdam Part. (2013); 73: 225–36.

Van Dongen H. P. et al., 'The cumulative cost of additional wakefulness: dose-response effects on neurobehavioral functions and sleep physiology from chronic sleep restriction and total sleep depriva-tion', *Sleep* (2003); 15, 26(2): 117–26.

Waters R. C., *So Built We the Wall*, Oxford: Hall the Printer Ltd., Littlegate (1937).

Waters R. C., *A Practice of Psychology*, George Allen and Unwin Ltd.

Waters R. C., 'Our thoughts affect our body's pre-sleep prep', *So Built We the Wall*, Oxford: Hall the Printer Ltd., Littlegate (1937), p118.

Chapter 1 – The Illusion of Impossibility

Alter D. S. and Sugarman L.I., 'Reorienting hypnosis education', *American Journal of Clinical Hypnosis* (2017); 59(3): 235–59.

Bargh J. A. and Chartrand T. L., 'The unbearable automaticity of being', *American Psychologist* (1999); 54(7): 462–79.

Braid J., 'Concentrated attention and various forms of suggestion', *The Discovery of Hypnosis. The complete writings of James Braid 'The Father of hypnotherapy'*, foreword by Dr Michael Heap, National Council for Hypnotherapy. Edited with commentary by Donald Robertson (p 237).

Coué É., *Self Mastery by Conscious Autosuggestion'*, the Lorraine Society of Applied Psychology (1921).

Coué, É., *How to Practice Suggestion and Autosuggestion*, American Library Service (1923).

Coué É. and Orton J. L., *Conscious Autosuggestion*, D. Appleton and Co. (1924).

Coué É., '[the unconscious mind] is credulous and accepts with unreasoning docility what it is told', *Self Mastery by Conscious Autosuggestion*, the Lorraine Society of Applied Psychology (1921), p 3.

Coué É., 'suspended from the summits of two cathedral towers': Coué É. and Orton J. L., *Conscious Autosuggestion* (1924), p 20.

Coué, É., 'Either way, we're "wretched puppets of which our imagina-tion holds all the strings." ' Coué É. *Self Mastery by Conscious*

Autosuggestion, the Lorraine Society of Applied Psychology (1921), p 7.

Coué, É., 'Contrary to what is taught …', Coué E., *Self Mastery by Conscious Autosuggestion*, the Lorraine Society of Applied Psychology (1921), p 92.

Ori Cohen, O. et al., 'Controlling an avatar by thought using real-time fMRI', *Journal of Neural Engineering* (2014); 11(3).

Corsetti M. and Whorwell P., 'The global impact of IBS: time to think about IBS-specific models of care?' *Therapeutic Advances in Gastroenterology* (2017); 10(9): 727–36.

Drew T., Vo M. L. H. and Wolfe J. M., 'The invisible gorilla strikes again: sustained inattentional blindness in expert observers', *Psychological Science* (2013); 24(9): 1848–53.

Elkins G., Jensen M. P. and Patterson D. R., 'Hypnotherapy for the management of chronic pain', *The International Journal of Clinical and Experimental Hypnosis* (2007); 55(3): 275–87.

Graci G. M. and Hardie J. C., 'Evidenced-based hypnotherapy for the management of sleep disorders', *Intl Journal of Clinical and Experimental Hypnosis* (2007); 55(3): 288–302.

Hardy J., Hall C. R. and Hardy L., 'Quantifying athlete self-talk', *Journal of Sports Sciences*, (2005); 23: 905–17.

Hope A. E. and Sugarman L. I., 'Orienting hypnosis', *American Journal of Clinical Hypnosis* (2015); 57(3): 212–29.

Dr Syed Shariq Hasan: interview with the author, July 2019.

Jenkins R. and Wiseman R., 'Darwin illusion: evolution in a blink of the eye', *Perception* (2009); 38(9): 1413–15.

Kaptchuk, T. J. and Miller, F. G., 'Placebo effects in medicine', *The New England Journal of Medicine* (2015); 373:1 nejm.org.

Kross, E. et al., 'Self-talk as a regulatory mechanism: how you do it matters', *Journal of Personality and Social Psychology* (2014); 106(2): 304–24.

Lam T., 'Hypnosis for insomnia: an exaggerated myth or an underrated intervention?' *Sleep Medicine*, Elsevier Science B.V., Amsterdam (2013); 14, SUPP/1: e176.

Kuhn G. and Land M.F., 'There's more to magic than meets the eye', *Current Biology* (2006); 16(22): R950–R951.

Macdonald K., executive mind coach and cognitive hypnotherapist: interview with the author, 22 April 2017.

Miller V., Carruthers H. R., Morris J., Hasan S. S., Archbold S. and Whorwell P. J., 'Hypnotherapy for irritable bowel syndrome: an audit of one thousand adult patients', *Aliment. Pharmacol. Ther.* (2015); 41(9): 844–55.

Miller V. and Whorwell P. J., 'Hypnotherapy for functional disorders', *A Review: International Journal of Clinical and Experimental Hypnosis* (2009); 57(3): 279–92.

Olson J. A. et al., 'Simulated thought insertion: influencing the sense of agency using deception and magic', *Consciousness and Cognition* (2016): 43: 11–26.

Sugarman L. I.: interview with the author, March 2018.

Sugarman L. I., 'Exploring, evolving, and refining hypnosis education', *American Journal of Clinical Hypnosis* (2017); 59(3): 231–32.

Sugarman L.I., 'Mapping the domain of hypnosis', *American Journal of Clinical Hypnosis*, (2015); 57(3): 209–11.

Tabibnia G. et al., 'The lasting effect of words on feelings: words may facilitate exposure effects to threatening images', *Emotion* (2008); 8(3): 307–17.

Thibault R. T., Veissière S., Olson J. A. and Raz A., 'Treating ADHD with suggestion: neurofeedback and placebo therapeutics', *Journal of Attention Disorders* (2018); 22(8): 707–11.

Thomas C. and Baker C. I., 'Teaching an adult brain new tricks: a critical review of evidence for training-dependent structural plasticity in humans', *NeuroImage*, Elsevier Science B.V., Amsterdam Part., (2013): 73: 225–236.

Tompkins M. L., *The Spectacle of Illusion: Magic, The Paranormal & The Complicity of The Mind*, Thames & Hudson Ltd (2019).

Vernillo A., 'Placebos in clinical practice and the power of suggestion', *American Journal of Bioethics* (2009); 9(12): 32–33.

Waters R. C. 'Émile Coué was the first to definitely link mind to matter', *So Built We the Wall,* Oxford: Hall the Printer Ltd., Littlegate (1937), (preface).

Wellcome Collection., 'Smoke and Mirrors: The Psychology of Magic', exhibition 2019.

Whorwell P. J., 'Hypnotherapy for irritable bowel syndrome: the response of colonic and noncolonic symptoms', *Journal of Psychosomatic Research* (2008); 64: 621–23.

Whorwell P. J. et al., 'Unexpected consequences: women's experiences of a self-hypnosis intervention to help with pain relief during labour', *Aliment. Pharmacol. Ther.* (2015); 41(9): 844–55.

Whorwell P, professor of medicine and gastroenterology at the Manchester University NHS Foundation Trust (MFT): interviews with the author, March 2018 and July 2019.

Williams L. E. and Bargh J. A., 'Experiencing physical warmth promotes interpersonal warmth', *Science* (2008); 322(5901): 606–07.

Wiseman R. and Greening E., 'It's still bending: verbal suggestion and alleged psychokinetic ability', *British Journal of Psychology* (2005); 96: 115–17.

Wolf T. H. et al., 'Effectiveness of self-hypnosis on the relief of experimental dental pain: a randomized trial', *The International Journal of Clinical and Experimental Hypnosis* Routledge, Taylor & Francis (2016); 64(2): 187–99.

Yapko M., 'Mindfulness and hypnosis: the power of suggestion to transform experience', *The American Journal of Clinical Hypnosis* (2012); 55(2): 199–200.

Chapter 2: Life Beneath Your Skin

American Academy of Sleep Medicine, *International Classification of Sleep Disorders,* 2nd ed, diagnostic and coding manual, Westchester, IL. (2005).

Cai D. J. et al., 'REM, not incubation, improves creativity by priming associative networks', *Proceedings of the National Academy of Sciences* (2009); 106(25): 10130–34.

Consensus Conference Panel: 'Recommended amount of sleep for a healthy adult: a joint consensus statement of the American Academy of Sleep Medicine and Sleep Research Society', *Sleep* (2015); 38(6):843–44.

Coué É., 'Everyone knows that the somnambulist gets up at night *without waking ...*', *Self Mastery by Conscious Autosuggestion*, (1921), p 2.

Ekirch A. R., *At Day's Close – A history of Nighttime*, W & N (2006).

Fleetham J. A. and Fleming J.A.: 'Parasomnias', *CMAJ* (2014);186(8): E273–80.

Fuller P. M., Gooley J, J. and Saper C. B., 'Neurobiology of the sleep–wake cycle: sleep architecture, circadian regulation, and regulatory feedback', *Journal of Biological Rhythms* (2006); 21(6): 482–93.

Hayashi M. et al., 'Recuperative power of a short daytime nap with or without Stage 2 sleep', *Sleep* (2005); 28(7): 829–36.

Herlin B. et al., 'Evidence that non-dreamers do dream: a REM sleep behaviour disorder model', *J. Sleep Res.* (2015); 24: 602–09.

Hobson J. A., 'Sleep is of the brain, by the brain and for the brain', *Nature* (2005); 437 (7063): 1254–6.

Kishi A. et al., 'NREM sleep stage transitions control ultradian REM sleep rhythm', *Sleep* (2011); 34(10): 1423–32.

Mednick S. et al., 'Sleep-dependent learning: a nap is as good as a night', *Nat. Neurosci.* (2003); 6(7): 697–8.

Naiman, R., 'Dreamless: the silent epidemic of REM sleep loss'. *Ann. N.Y. Acad. Sci.* (2017); 1406: 77–85.

Orton J. L., 'But though the idea was abandoned so far as Coué himself was concerned, the Maharajah took other steps to assist in the spread of Couéism': Émile Coué: The Man and His Work, (1935), p192.

Popat S. and Winslade W., 'While you were sleepwalking: science and neurobiology of sleep disorders & the enigma of legal responsibility of violence during parasomnia', *Neuroethics* (2015); 8(2): 203–14.

Reichert S., Arocas O. P. and Rihel R. J., 'The neuropeptide galanin is required for homeostatic rebound sleep following increased neuronal activity', *Neuron*. (2019).

The Sleep Council, The Great British Bedtime Report (2013 and 2017): www.sleepcouncil.org.uk.

Stranges S. et al., 'Cross-sectional versus prospective associations of sleep duration with changes in relative weight and body fat distribution: the Whitehall II Study', *American Journal of Epidemiology* (2008); 167(3): 321–9.

Waters R. C., 'Sleep is not rest if rest is understood as inertia or idleness …': *So Built We the Wall*. Oxford: Hall the Printer Ltd., Littlegate (1937), p 118.

Waters R. C., 'We explain to the patient the cause and nature of his trouble…': *So Built We the Wall*. Oxford: Hall the Printer Ltd., Littlegate (1937), p 52.

Waters R.C., 'Our endocrine system – our glands and their hormones – are who we are, affecting our personality "to an extraordinary extent"': *So Built We the Wall*. Oxford: Hall The Printer Ltd., Littlegate (1937), p 26.

Zhu Y. et al., 'Degeneration in arousal neurons in chronic sleep disruption modeling sleep apnea', *Frontiers in Neurology* (2015); 6: 109.

Zhu Y. et al., 'Intermittent short sleep results in lasting sleep wake disturbances and degeneration of locus coeruleus and orexinergic neurons', *Sleep* (2016); 39(8): 1601–11.

Chapter 3: The Big Primordial Tick Tock

American Medical Association., 'AMA adopts guidance to reduce harm from high intensity street lights' (2016).

Bank of America Trends in Consumer Mobility Report (2015).

Baron K. G. and Reid K. J., 'Circadian misalignment and health', *International Review of Psychiatry,* Abingdon, England (2014); 26(2): 139–54.

Born J., Hansen K., Marshall L., Mölle M., Fehm H.: 'Timing the End of Nocturnal Sleep', *Nature* (1999); 397: 29–30.

Boubekri M. et al., 'The Impact of optimized daylight and views on the sleep duration and cognitive performance of office workers', *Int. J. Environ. Res. Public Health* (2020); 17: 3219.

Dr George Brainard: interview with the author, 29 March 2018.

Brainard G. C. et al., 'Action spectrum for melatonin regulation in humans: evidence for a novel circadian photoreceptor', *The Journal of Neuroscience* (2001); 21(16): 6405–12.

Brainard G. C. et al., 'The development of lighting countermeasures for sleep disruption and circadian misalignment during spaceflight', *Wolters Kluwer Health, Inc.* (2016); 22.

Cassone V. M. and Westneat D. F., 'The bird of time: cognition and the avian biological clock', *Frontiers in Molecular Neuroscience* (2012); 5: 32.

Chang A. M., et al., 'Impact of light-emitting ebooks before bed', *Proceedings of the National Academy of Sciences* (2015); 112(4): 1232–37.

Duffy J. F. and Czeisler C. A., 'Effect of light on human circadian physiology', *Sleep Medicine Clinics* (2009); 4(2): 165–77.

Exelmans L. and Van den Bulck J., 'Binge viewing, sleep, and the role of pre-sleep arousal', *Journal of Clinical Sleep Medicine: JCSM : Official Publication of the American Academy of Sleep Medicine* (2017); 13(8): 1001–08.

Fuller P. M., Lu J. and Saper C.B., 'Differential rescue of light-and food-entrainable circadian rhythms', *Science* (2008); 320: 1074–77.

Glickman G., Byrne B., Pineda C., Hauck W. W. and Brainard G. C., 'Light therapy for seasonal affective disorder with blue narrow-band light-emitting diodes (LEDs)', *Biological Psychiatry* (2006); 9: 502–07.

Grubisic M. et al., 'Insect declines and agroecosystems: does light pollution matter?' *Annals of Applied Biology* (2018); 173: 180–89.

Huang W. et al. 'Circadian Rhythms, Sleep, and Metabolism', *J. Clin. Invest.* (2011); 121(6): 2133–41.

Ibáñez C., 'Scientific background discoveries of molecular mechanisms controlling the circadian rhythm', The Nobel Assembly at Karolinska Institutet (2017).

Kuss D. J. et al., 'Problematic mobile phone use and addiction across generations: the roles of psychopathological symptoms and smartphone use', J. Technol. Behav. Sci. (2018); 3: 141–9.

Marqueze E. C. et al., 'Natural light exposure, sleep and depression among day workers and shiftworkers at Arctic and Equatorial latitudes', PLoS ONE (2015); 10(4): e0122078.

McClung C. R., 'Plant circadian rhythms', The Plant Cell (2006);18(4): 792–803.

McElvenny D. M. et al., 'What should we tell shift workers to do to reduce their cancer risk?', Occupational Medicine (2018); 68(1): 5–7.

Najjar R. P. et al., 'Chronic artificial blue-enriched white light is an effective countermeasure to delayed circadian phase and neurobehavioral decrements', PLoS ONE (2014); 9(7): e102827.

National Sleep Foundation, International Bedroom Poll, 2013.

Patel S. R. and Hu F. B., 'Short sleep duration and weight gain: a systematic review', Obesity (Silver Spring) (2008); 16: 643–53.

Rod N. H. et al., 'Overnight smartphone use: a new public health challenge? A novel study design based on high-resolution smartphone data', PLoS One (2018);13(10): e0204811.

Sandhu A., Seth M. and Gurm H. S., 'Daylight savings time and myocardial infarction', Open Heart (2014); 1(1): e000019.

Stevens R. G. and Brainard G. C. et al., 'Breast cancer and circadian disruption from electric lighting in the modern world', CA Cancer J. Clin. (2014); 64: 207–18.

Tonsfeldt K. J. and Chappell P. E., 'Clocks on top: the role of the circadian clock in the hypothalamic and pituitary regulation of endocrine physiology', Molecular and Cellular Endocrinology (2012); 349(1): 3–12.

Wittmann M. et al., 'Social jetlag: misalignment of biological and social time', Chronobiology International (2009); 23(1–2): 497–509.

Chapter 4: A Carrot for Your Habit – How
to Create Positives for Sleep

Bargh J. A. and Chartrand T. L., 'The unbearable automaticity of being', *American Psychologist* (1999); 54(7): 462–79.

Coué É., 'It is impossible to think of two things at once': *Self Mastery by Conscious Autosuggestion*, p 13.

Coué É., 'Every idea that we put into the mind becomes a reality in so far as it is within the realms of possibility ...': *How to Practice Suggestion and Autosuggestion*, p 59.

Coué E., 'How is one to explain to oneself and to explain to others that the repetition of the same words "I am going to sleep ..."': *Self Mastery by Conscious Autosuggestion*, p 90.

Graybiel A. M. and Smith K. S., 'Good habits, bad habits. Researchers are pinpointing the brain circuits that can help us form good habits and break bad ones', *Scientific American* (2014); 310: 38–43.

Lally P. et al., 'How are habits formed: modelling habit formation in the real world', *Eur. J. Soc. Psychol.* (2010); 40: 998–1009.

Neal D. T., Wood W., Wu M. and Kurlander D., 'The pull of the past: when do habits persist despite conflict with motives?' *Personality and Social Psychology Bulletin* (2011); 37(11): 1428.

Neal D. T. et al., 'How do habits guide behaviour? Perceived and actual triggers of habits in daily life', *Journal of Experimental Social Psychology* (2012); 48: 492–8.

Orton J. L., 'The roadway to where he stayed was lined with limousines and perambulators, bath chairs and sick beds': Émile Coué: The Man and His Work (1935) l, p107.

Savani K. and Job V., 'Reverse ego-depletion: acts of self-control can improve subsequent performance in Indian cultural contexts', *Journal of Personality and Social Psychology* (2017); 113(4): 589–607.

Smith K. S. and Graybiel A. M. 'Investigating habits: strategies, technologies and models', *Frontiers in Behavioral Neuroscience* (2014); 8: 39.

Dr Kyle S. Smith: interview with the author, 13 March 2018.

Smith K. S. and Graybiel A. M., 'Habit formation coincides with shifts in reinforcement representations in the sensorimotor striatum', *J. Neurophysiol.* (2016); 115: 1487–98.

Smith K. S. and Graybiel A. M., 'Habit formation', *Dialogues in Clinical Neuroscience* (2016); 18(1): 33–43.

Waters R. C., 'The amount of impression which we can obtain by one direct suggestion is limited . . .', *A Practice of Psychology*, p 35.

Wood W., Quinn J. M. and Kashy D. A., 'Habits in everyday life: thought, emotion, and action', *Journal of Personality and Social Psychology. The American Psychological Association, Inc.* (2002); 83(6): 1281–97 0022–3514.

Chapter 5: How Do You Feel Exactly?
Give it a Name. Any. Name. You. Like.

Baumeister R.F., Bratslavsky E., Finkenauer C. and Vohs K. D., 'Bad is stronger than good'. *Review of General Psychology* (2001); 5(4): 323–70.

Ben-Simon E. and Walker M. P., 'Sleep loss causes social withdrawal and loneliness', *Nat. Commun.* (2018); 9: 3146.

Black D. S., O'Reilly G.A., Olmstead R., et al. 'Mindfulness meditation and improvement in sleep quality and daytime impairment among older adults with sleep disturbances: a randomized clinical trial', *JAMA Intern. Med.* (2015); 22(4).

Brianza G., et al., 'As light as your scent: effects of smell and sound on body image perception', International Conference on Human-Computer Interaction (2019).

Brooks A.W., 'Get excited: reappraising pre-performance anxiety as excitement', *Journal of Experimental Psychology: General* (2014); 143(3): 1144–58.

Brooks, Alison Wood: interview with the author, 9 March 2018.

Brooks A. W., Schroeder J., et al., 'Don't stop believing: rituals improve performance by decreasing anxiety', *Organizational Behavior and Human Decision Processes* (2016); 137: 71–85.

Bushdid C., et al. 'Humans can discriminate more than 1 trillion olfactory stimuli', *Science* (2014); 343 (6177): 1370–2.

Cacioppo S. et al., 'Loneliness: clinical import and interventions', *Perspectives on Psychological Science: a journal of the Association for Psychological Science* (2015); 10(2): 238–49.

Creswell J. D. et al., 'Mindfulness-Based Stress Reduction training reduces loneliness and pro-inflammatory gene expression in older adults: a small randomized controlled trial', *Brain, Behavior, and Immunity* (2012); 26(7): 1095–101.

Dodge R., Daly A., Huyton J. and Sanders L., 'The challenge of defining wellbeing', *International Journal of Wellbeing* (2012); 2(3): 222–35.

Dong S. and Jacob T. J. C., 'Combined non-adaptive light and smell stimuli lowered blood pressure, reduced heart rate and reduced negative affect', *Physiology & Behavior* (2016); 156: 94–105.

Professor Robin Dunbar: interview with the author, 24 March 2020.

Feldman Barrett L. *How Emotions Are Made*, Pan (2017).

Feldman Barrett L. 'The science of emotion: what people believe, what the evidence shows, and where to go from here' National Research Council, *Human Behavior in Military Contexts*, Washington, DC: The National Academies Press (2008).

Hardy J. and Oliver E. J., 'Self-talk, positive thinking, and thought stopping', *Encyclopedia of Sport and Exercise Psychology*, Thousand Oaks, California: Sage (2014).

Hawkley L. C. and Cacioppo J. T., 'Loneliness matters: a theoretical and empirical review of consequences and mechanisms', *Annals of Behavioral Medicine: a Publication of the Society of Behavioral Medicine* (2010); 40(2): 218–27.

Hershfield H. E. et al., 'When feeling bad can be good: mixed emotions benefit physical health across adulthood', *Social Psychological and Personality Science* (2013); 4(1): 54–61.

Kaptchuk T. J. and Miller F. G., 'Placebo effects in medicine', *The New England Journal of Medicine* (2015); 373: 8–9.

Killingsworth M. A. and Gilbert D. T., 'A wandering mind is an unhappy mind', *Science* (2010); 330(6006): 932.

Kok B. E., Coffey KA. et al., 'How positive emotions build physical health: perceived positive social connections account for the upward spiral between positive emotions and vagal tone' *Psychological Science* (2013); 24. 10.1177.

Larsen J. T., Hemenover S. H., Norris C. J. and Cacioppo J. T., 'Turning adversity to advantage: on the virtues of the coactivation of positive and negative emotions', *A Psychology of Human Strengths: Perspectives on an Emerging Field,* Washington, DC: *American Psychological Association* (2003); 211–26.

Lim N., 'Cultural differences in emotion: differences in emotional arousal level between the east and the west', *Integrative Medicine Research* (2016); 5(2): 105–09.

Dr Tim Lomas: interview with the author, 12 March 2018.

Lomas T. 'Ambivalent emotions: a cross-cultural conceptual review of their relevance to wellbeing', School of Psychology, University of East London (2018).

Lomas T.: 'The flavours of love: a cross-cultural lexical analysis'. *J. Theory. Soc. Behav.* (2018); 48: 134–52.

Masi C. M., Chen H. Y., Hawkley L. C. and Cacioppo J. T., 'A meta-analysis of interventions to reduce loneliness', *Personality and Social Psychology Review: an Official Journal of the Society for Personality and Social Psychology, Inc.* (2010); 15(3): 219–66.

Norton M. I. and Gino F., 'Rituals alleviate grieving for loved ones, lovers, and lotteries', *Journal of Experimental Psychology: General* (2014); 143: 266–72.

Sánchez-Vidaña D. I. et al., 'The effectiveness of aromatherapy for depressive symptoms: a systematic review', *Evidence-based Complementary and Alternative Medicine: eCAM* (2017); 2017: 5869315.

Simon B. E. et al., 'Losing neutrality: the neural basis of impaired emotional control without sleep', *Journal of Neuroscience* (2015); 35: 13194–13205.

University of Sussex, 'As light as a lemon: how the right smell can help with a negative body image'. *ScienceDaily* (2019).

de Wijk R. A. and Zijlstra S. M., 'Differential effects of exposure to ambient vanilla and citrus aromas on mood, arousal and food choice', *Flavour* (2012); 1: 24.

Winbush N. Y., Gross C. R. and Kreitzer M. J., 'The effects of Mindfulness-Based Stress Reduction on sleep disturbance: a systematic review', *The Journal of Science & Healing* (2007); 3(6): 585–91.

Wolf E. B., Lee J. J., Sah S. and Brooks A.W., 'Managing perceptions of distress at work: reframing emotion as passion', *Organizational Behavior and Human Decision Processes* (2016); 137: 1–12

Chapter 6: Slow Down, You're Moving Too Fast

Adler R. F. and Benbunan-Fich R., 'The effects of task difficulty and multitasking on performance', *Interacting with Computers* (2015); 27, 4(1): 430–39.

American Psychological Association, 'Stress in America. Coping with Change', 2017 and 2020.

Basta M. et al., 'Chronic insomnia and stress system', *Sleep Medicine Clinics* (2007); 2(2): 279–91.

Baumeister R. F. et al., 'Bad is stronger than good', *Review of General Psychology* (2001); 5(4): 323–70.

Bavishi A., Slade M. D. and Levy B. R., 'A chapter a day: association of book reading with longevity', *Social Science & Medicine* (2016); 164: 44–48.

Buric I. et al., 'What is the molecular signature of mind–body interventions? A systematic review of gene expression changes induced by meditation and related practices', *Frontiers in Immunology* (2017); 8: 670.

Carney D. R., Cuddy A. J. C. and Yap A. J., 'Power posing: brief non-verbal displays affect neuroendocrine levels and risk tolerance', *Psychological Science* (2010); 1363–68.

Coué É., 'No, that does not trouble me at all': Self Mastery by Conscious Autosuggestion (1921); p67.

Crum A., Salovey P. and Achor S., 'Rethinking stress: the role of mindsets in determining the stress response' *Journal of Personality and Social Psychology* (2013); 104: 727.

Crum A. and Lyddy C., 'De-stressing stress: the power of mindsets and the art of stressing mindfully', *The Wiley Blackwell Handbook of Mindfulness* (2014); 1–2: 948–63.

Crum A. J. and Langer E. J., 'Mind-set matters: exercise and the placebo effect', *Psychological Science* (2007);18(2): 165–71.

Crum A., 'Gladstone rethinks stress with mindset expert Alia Crum', Youtube, 2016.

Cuddy A. J. C., 'Your body language may shape who you are', Ted Talk, 2012.

Cuddy A. J. C., Schultz S. J. and Fosse N. E., 'P-Curving a more comprehensive body of research on postural feedback reveals clear evidential value for power-posing effects: reply to Simmons and Simonsohn 2017', *Psychological Science* (2018); 29(4): 656–66.

Emmons R. A. and McCullough D. M. E., 'Counting blessings versus burdens: an experimental investigation of gratitude and subjective well-being in daily life', *Journal of Personality and Social Psychology* (2003); 84(2): 377–89.

The European Environment Agency: Noise in Europe 2014. EEA Report No 10/2014.

The European Environment Agency: Environmental Noise in Europe 2020. EEA Report No 22/ 2019.

Galinsky A. and Kilduff G. J., 'Be seen as a leader', *Harvard Business Review* (2013).

Hammond C. and Lewis G., 'The rest test: preliminary findings from a large-scale international survey on rest', *The Restless Compendium: Interdisciplinary Investigations of Rest and Its Opposites* (2016); Chapter 8.

The Harvard Study of Adult Development: https://www.adultdevelopmentstudy.org/

International Labour Organization: 'Workplace Stress: A Collective Challenge' (2016).

Kalyani B. G., Venkatasubramanian G., Arasappa R. et al., 'Neurohemodynamic correlates of 'OM' chanting: a pilot functional magnetic resonance imaging study'. *International Journal of Yoga* (2011); 4(1): 3–6.

'Reading a paper book cuts stress by up to 68 per cent', Lewis D., Galaxy Stress Research. Mindlab International, Sussex University, UK. 2009.

Li Q., Morimoto K., Kobayashi M. et al., 'Visiting a forest, but not a city, increases human natural killer activity and expression of anti-cancer proteins'. *International Journal of Immunopathology and Pharmacology* (2008); 117–27.

Li Q. et al., 'Effect of phytoncide from trees on human natural killer cell function', *International Journal of Immunopathology and Pharmacology* (2009); 22(4): 951–59.

Lobo V., Patil A., Phatak A. and Chandra N., 'Free radicals, antioxidants and functional foods: impact on human health', *Pharmacogn. Rev.* (2010); 4 (8): 118–26.

Malone J. C., Cohen S., Liu S. R., Vaillant G. E., Waldinger R. J., 'Adaptive midlife defense mechanisms and late-life health', *Pers. Individ. Dif.* (2013); 55(2): 85–89.

McKinney M. D. et al., 'The health benefits of physical activity and cardiorespiratory fitness', *BCMJ.* (2016); 58(3): 131–37.

Michalak, J., Mischnat, J. and Teismann, T., 'Sitting posture makes a difference – embodiment effects on depressive memory bias'. *J. Investig. Psych. Offender Profil.* (2014); 21: 519–24.

Miller G. A., 'The magical number seven, plus or minus two some limits on our capacity for processing information'. *The American Psychological Association. Psychological Review* (1955); 101(2): 343–52.

Morita E., et al., 'Psychological effects of forest environments on healthy adults: Shinrin-yoku (forest-air bathing, walking) as a possible method of stress reduction', *Public Health* (2007); 121(1): 54–63.

Murtagh E. M., Murphy M. H. and Boone-Heinonen J. 'Walking – the First Steps in Cardiovascular Disease Prevention', *Current Opinion in Cardiology* (2010); 25(5): 490–96.

Nelson-Coffey S. et al., 'Do unto others or treat yourself? The effects of prosocial and self-focused behavior on psychological flourishing', *Emotion* (2016); 16.

Nutt D., Wilson S. and Paterson L., 'Sleep disorders as core symptoms of depression', *Dialogues Clin. Neurosci.* (2008); 10(3): 329–36.

Park B. J. et al., 'The physiological effects of *Shinrin-yoku* (taking in the forest atmosphere or forest bathing): evidence from field experiments in 24 forests across Japan', *Environmental Health and Preventive Medicine* (2010); 15(1): 18–26.

Passos G. S. et al., 'Is Exercise an alternative treatment for chronic insomnia?', *Clinics* (2012); 67(6): 653–59.

Robertson I. H., 'The stress test: can stress ever be beneficial?', *Journal of The British Academy* (2017); 5: 163–76.

Schiff, B. B. and M Lamon., 'Inducing emotion by unilateral contraction of hand muscles', *Cortex* (1994); 30(2): 247–54.

Sliter M., Kale A. and Yuan Z., 'Is humor the best medicine? The buffering effect of coping humor on traumatic stressors in firefighters', *J. Organiz. Behav.* (2014); 35: 257–72.

Tops M. and De Jong R.: 'Posing for success: clenching a fist facilitates approach', *Psychonomic Bulletin & Review* (2006); 13: 229–34.

Tsunetsugu Y., Park B-J. and Miyazaki Y., 'Trends in research related to 'Shinrin-yoku' (taking in the forest atmosphere or forest bathing) in Japan'. *Environmental Health and Preventive Medicine* (2010); 15(1): 27–37.

Tyrväinen L. et al., 'The influence of urban green environments on stress relief measures: a field experiment'. *Journal of Environmental Psychology* (2014); 38: 1–9.

Uvnäs-Moberg K., Handlin L. and Petersson M., 'Self-soothing behaviors with particular reference to oxytocin release induced by non-noxious sensory stimulation', *Frontiers in Psychology* (2015); 5: 1529.

Villarroel H. S. et al., 'NPY induces stress resilience via downregu-lation of *I*h in principal neurons of rat basolateral amygdala', *Journal of Neuroscience* (2018); 38(19): 4505–20.

Waters R. C., 'Let us suppose now that fear is active in the mind . . .': Waters R. C., *A Practice of Psychology*, George Allen and Unwin Ltd. p20.

Waters R. C., 'Tonight, as soon as I decide to go to bed': *So built We the Wall*. Oxford: Hall the Printer Ltd., Littlegate (1937), (Insomnia, p120)

Webb C: *How to Have a Good Day*, Pan (2016).

World Health Organization: https://www.who.int/en/news-room/fact-sheets/detail/depression

Young S. N., 'How to increase serotonin in the human brain without drugs', *Journal of Psychiatry & Neuroscience: JPN* (2007); 32(6): 394–99.

Zahrt O. H., Crum A. J., 'Perceived physical activity and mor-tality: evidence from three nationally representative U.S. samples' *Health Psychology* (2017); 36(11): 1017–25.

Chapter 7: The Invisible Rollercoaster – What and When We Eat Matters

Bravo R. et al., 'Tryptophan-enriched cereal intake improves nocturnal sleep, melatonin, serotonin, and total antioxidant capacity levels and mood in elderly humans', *AGE* (2013); 35(4): 1277–85.

Briguglio M. et al., 'Dietary neurotransmitters: a narrative review on current knowledge', *Nutrients* (2018); 10(5): 591.

Dr Eugene Chang: interview with the author, March 2018.

Chaput J. P., Després J. P., Bouchard C. and Tremblay A., 'Short sleep duration is associated with reduced leptin levels and increased adiposity: results from the Quebec family study', *Obesity* (2007); 15: 253–61.

Chaput J. P., Després J. P., Bouchard C. and Tremblay A., 'The associ-ation between sleep duration and weight gain in adults: a 6-year prospective study from the Quebec family study'. *Sleep* (2008); 31(4): 517–23

Crum A. et al., 'Mind Over milkshakes: mindsets, not just nutrients, determine ghrelin response', *Health Psychology* (2011); 30(4): 424–29.

Djokic G. et al., 'The effects of magnesium – melatonin – vit B complex supplementation in treatment of insomnia', *Open Access Maced. J. Med. Sci.* (2019); 7(18): 3101–05.

Fonken L. K. et al., 'Light at night increases body mass by shifting the time of food intake', *Proceedings of the National Academy of Sciences of the United States of America* (2010); 107(43): 18664–69.

Grandner M. A., Jackson N., Gerstner J. R., Knutson K. L., 'Sleep symptoms associated with intake of specific dietary nutrients', *Journal of Sleep Research* (2014); 23(1): 22–34.

Howatson G. et al., 'Effect of tart cherry juice (*prunus cerasus*) on melatonin levels and enhanced sleep quality', *Eur. J. Nutr.* (2012); 51(8): 909–16.

Ileri-Gurel E., Pehlivanoglu B. and Dogan M., 'Effect of acute stress on taste perception: in relation with baseline anxiety level and body weight', *Chemical Senses* (2013); 38(1): 27–34.

Jenkins T.A. et al., 'Influence of tryptophan and serotonin on mood and cognition with a possible role of the gut-brain axis', *Nutrients* (2016); 8(1): 56.

Kim S. et al., 'GABA and l-theanine mixture decreases sleep latency and improves NREM sleep', *Pharmaceutical Biology* (2019); 57(1): 64–72.

Kinsey A. W., Ormsbee M. J., 'The health impact of nighttime eating: old and new perspectives', *Nutrients* (2015); 7(4): 2648–62.

Kohsaka A. et al., 'High-fat diet disrupts behavioral and molecular circadian rhythms in mice', *Cell Metabolism* (2007); 6(5): 414–21.

Linares I. M. P. et al., 'No acute effects of cannabidiol on the sleep–wake cycle of healthy subjects: a randomized, double-blind, placebo-controlled, crossover study', *Front. Pharmacol.* (2018); 9: 315.

Markwald R. R. et al., 'Insufficient sleep and weight gain', *Proceedings of the National Academy of Sciences* (2013); 110(14): 5695–700.

Monda V., Villano I. and Messina A. et al., 'Exercise modifies the gut microbiota with positive health effects', *Oxidative Medicine and Cellular Longevity* (2017); volume article ID 3831972: 8.

Ness K. M. et al., 'Four nights of sleep restriction suppress the post-prandial lipemic response and decrease satiety', *Journal of Lipid Research* (2019); 60: 1935–45.

Oike H., Oishi K. and Kobori M., 'Nutrients, clock genes, and chron-onutrition' *Current Nutrition Reports* (2014); 3(3): 204–12.

Orton J. L: Émile Coué: The Man and His Work (1935).

Pejovic S., et al., 'Leptin and hunger levels in young healthy adults after one night of sleep loss', *Journal of Sleep Research* (2010); 19: 552–58.

Perkins S: Interview with the author, March 2018.

Potter G. D. M. et al., 'Circadian rhythm and sleep disruption: causes, metabolic consequences, and countermeasures', *Endocrine Reviews* (2016); 37(6): 584–608.

Renzella J. et al., 'What national and subnational interventions and policies based on Mediterranean and Nordic diets are recommended or implemented in the WHO European region, and is there evidence of effectiveness in reducing noncommunicable diseases?', *World Health Organization*, 2018.

Shannon S., Lewis N., Lee H. and Hughes S., 'Cannabidiol in anxiety and sleep: a large case series', *Perm. J.* (2019); 23: 18-041.

Taheri S., et al.: 'Short sleep duration is associated with reduced leptin, elevated ghrelin, and increased body mass index', *PLoS Med.* (2004); 1(3): e62.

Thompson R. S. et al., 'Dietary prebiotics and bioactive milk fractions improve NREM sleep, enhance REM sleep rebound and attenuate the stress-induced decrease in diurnal temperature and gut microbial alpha diversity', *Front. Behav. Neurosci.* (2017); 10: 240.

Wheatley D., 'Medicinal plants for insomnia: a review of their pharmacology, efficacy and tolerability', *J. Psychopharmacol.* (2005); 19: 414–21.

Zeng Y., Yang J. and Du J. et al., 'Strategies of functional foods promote sleep in human being', *Current Signal Transduction Therapy* (2014); 9(3): 148–55.

Chapter 8: Feeling Flush

Alexander C. N., Langer E. J., *Higher Stages of Human Development*, Oxford University Press, 1990.

Ayers B. et al., 'The impact of attitudes towards the menopause on women's symptom experience: a systematic review', *Maturitas* (2010); 65(1): 28–36.

Baker F, C., de Zambotti M., Colrain I. M. and Bei B., 'Sleep problems during the menopausal transition: prevalence, impact, and management challenges', *Nature and Science of Sleep* (2018); 10: 73–95.

British Menopause Society; thebms.org.uk.

Dalal P. K. and Agarwal M., 'Postmenopausal Syndrome', *Indian Journal of Psychiatry* (2015); 57(2): S222–32.

Draper C. F. et al., 'Menstrual cycle rhythmicity: metabolic patterns in healthy women', *Scientific Reports* (2018); 8(1): 14568.

Driver H. S. et al., 'The menstrual cycle effects on sleep', *Sleep Medicine Clinics* (2008); 3;(1): 1–12.

Dunneram Y. et al., 'Dietary intake and age at natural menopause: results from the UK Women's Cohort Study', *J. Epidemiol. Community Health* (2018); 72: 733–40.

Franco O. H., Chowdhury R., Troup J. et al., 'Use of plant-based therapies and menopausal symptoms: a systematic review and meta-analysis', *JAMA* (2016); 315(23): 2554–63.

Hunter M. et al., 'Prevalence, frequency and problem rating of hot flushes persist in older postmenopausal women: impact of age, body mass index, hysterectomy, hormone therapy use, lifestyle and mood in a cross-sectional cohort study of 10,418 British women aged 54–65', *BJOG* (2012); 119: 40–50.

Hunter M. and Smith M., *Managing Hot Flushes and Night Sweats. A Cognitive Behavioural Self-Help Guide to the Menopause*, Routledge (2014).

Husain D. et al., 'Supplementation of soy isoflavones improved sex hormones, blood pressure, and postmenopausal symptoms', *Journal of the American College of Nutrition* (2015); 34(1): 42–48.

Im E. O., 'Ethnic differences in symptoms experienced during the menopausal transition', *Health Care for Women International* (2009); 30(4): 339–55.

Kowalcek I. et al., 'Women's attitude and perceptions towards menopause in different cultures: cross-cultural and intra-cultural comparison of pre-menopausal and post-menopausal women in Germany and in Papua New Guinea', *Maturitas* (2005); 51(3): 227–35.

Kravitz H. M. et al., 'Sleep disturbance during the menopausal transition in a multi-ethnic community sample of women', *Sleep* (2008); 31(7): 979–90.

Langer E. J., *Counter Clockwise: Mindful health and the Power of Possibility*, Ballantine Books, NY (2009).

Levy B. R., 'Mind matters: cognitive and physical effects of aging self-stereotypes', *The Journals of Gerontology: Series B* (2003); 58(4): 203–11.

Levy B. R., Slade M. D. and Kasl S. V., 'Longitudinal benefit of positive self-perceptions of aging on functional health', *The Journals of Gerontology: Series B* (2002); 57(5): 409–17.

Pagnini F. and Langer E. et al., 'Ageing as a mindset: a study protocol to rejuvenate older adults with a counterclockwise psychological intervention', *BMJ Open* (2019); 9(7): e030411.

Dr Mary Jane Minkin: interview with author, 18 February 2019.

Minkin M. J.: http://madameovary.com/

Murphy P. J. and Campbell S. S., 'Sex hormones, sleep, and core body temperature in older postmenopausal women', *Sleep* (2007); 30(12): 1788–94.

National Institutes of Health, 'Sleep problems during the menopausal transition' (2018).

National Sleep Foundation: www.sleepfoundation.org

Shechter A. and Boivin, D. B., 'Sleep, hormones, and circadian rhythms throughout the menstrual cycle in healthy women and women with premenstrual dysphoric disorder', *International Journal of Endocrinology* (2010); 259345.

Sood R. et al., 'Paced breathing compared with usual breathing for hot flashes, menopause', *The Journal of the North American Menopause Society* (2013); 20(2): 179–84.

Tonick S. and Muneyyirci-Delale O., 'Magnesium in women's health and gynecology', *Open Journal of Obstetrics and Gynecology* (2016); 6: 325–33.

de Zambotti M. et al., 'Menstrual cycle-related variation in physiological sleep in women in the early menopausal transition, *The Journal of Clinical Endocrinology & Metabolism* (2015); 100(8): 2918–26.

Chapter 9: Are You Listening Carefully?

Coué É., 'the simplest thing in the world': Coué É.: *Self Mastery by Conscious Autosuggestion* (1921), p 13.

Coué É., 'Because it is too easy to understand! There are those who cannot imagine so simple a thing will produce such an effect!', *How to Practice Suggestion and Autosuggestion* (1923), p 44.

Dr Syed Shariq Hasan: interview with the author, 16 July 2019.

Kirsty Macdonald: interview with author, 22 April 2017.

Waters R. C., ''Tonight, as soon as I decide to go to bed, my sense of the realisation of bed time will be followed by strong and sustained action throughout my system', *So Built We the Wall*. Oxford: Hall the Printer Ltd., Littlegate (1937), p 120.

Waters R. C., 'An excellent time to train this suggestion into the mind …': *So Built We the Wall*. Oxford: Hall the Printer Ltd., Littlegate (1937), p 120.

Waters R. C., 'The amount of impression which we can obtain by one direct suggestion is limited …': *A Practice of Psychology*, p35.

Chapter 10: From the Outside In

Ali B. et al., 'Essential oils used in aromatherapy: a systemic review', *Asian Pacific Journal of Tropical Biomedicine* (2015); 5(8): 601–11.

Baron K. G. et al., 'Orthosomnia: are some patients taking the quantified self too far?', *Journal of Clinical Sleep Medicine: JCSM : official publication of the American Academy of Sleep Medicine* (2017); 13(2): 351–54.

Chiba S. et al., 'High rebound mattress toppers facilitate core body temperature drop and enhance deep sleep in the initial phase of nocturnal sleep', *PLoS One* (2018); 13(6): e0197521.

Goes T. C. et al., 'Effect of sweet orange aroma on experimental anxiety in humans', *The Journal of Alternative and Complementary Medicine* (2012); 18(8): 798–804.

Hsieh T.H. et al., 'The tent-type clean unit system platform for air cleaning and non-contact sleep assessment. In proceedings of the 2019 3rd International Conference on Computational Biology and Bioinformatics (ICCBB 2019)', *Association for Computing Machinery, New York*, (2019); 47–51.

Karadag E. et al., 'Effects of aromatherapy on sleep quality and anxiety of patients', *Nurs. Crit. Care* (2017); 22: 105–12.

Khayat R. N. and Jafari B., 'Snoring in the morning light', *J. Clin. Sleep Med.* (2016); 12 (12): 1581–82.

Rao N. G. et al., 'Effect of a novel photoelectrochemical oxidation air purifier on nasal and ocular allergy symptoms', *Allergy Rhinol.* (2018); 9: 2152656718781609.

Resta O. et al., 'Sleep-related breathing disorders, loud snoring and excessive daytime sleepiness in obese subjects', *International Journal of Obesity* (2001); 25: 669–75.

Riedy S. M. et al., 'Noise as a sleep aid: a systematic review', *Sleep Medicine Reviews* (2021); 55: 101385.

Shin M. et al., 'The effects of fabric for sleepwear and bedding on sleep at ambient temperatures of 17°C and 22°C', *Nat. Sci. Sleep* (2016); 8: 121–31.

Sleep Council's Great British Bedtime Report. 2013 & 2017: www. sleepcouncil.org.uk.

Sublett J. L., 'Effectiveness of air filters and air cleaners in allergic respiratory diseases: a review of the recent literature', *Curr. Allergy Asthma Rep.* (2011); 11: 395.

Svanborg, E., et al., 'Snoring causes OSA: sensory nervous lesions in the palate worsen over time in untreated snorers but not in CPAP-treated patients', *Journal of Sleep Research* (2018); 27(1): 399.

Svensson M. et al., 'Daytime sleepiness relates to snoring independent of the apnea-hypopnea Index in women from the general population', *Chest* (2008); 134(5): 919–24.

Chapter 11: The Protégé with a Crystal Ball

Andrillon T. et al., 'Neural markers of responsiveness to the environment in human sleep', *Journal of Neuroscience* (2016); 36(24): 6583–96.

McBlain M., Jones K.A., Shannon G., 'Sleeping Eurasian oystercatchers adjust their vigilance in response to the behaviour of neighbours, human disturbance and environmental conditions', *J. Zool.* (2020); 312: 75–84.

Cirelli C. and Tononi G., 'Is sleep essential?', *PLoS Biol.* (2008); 6 (8): e216.

Coué É., 'The idea of sleep creates sleep; the idea of sleeplessness creates sleeplessness. What is a person who sleeps well? It is a person who knows that when one is in the bed it is for sleep, and he sleeps.': *How to Practice Suggestion and Autosuggestion* (1923): p 111

Coué É.: www.congresmethodecoue.com.

Durupt F., 'Mais Finalement, Quelle est la Méthode de la Méthode Coué?' *Liberation* (11 October 2017).

Hendricks J. C et al., 'Rest in drosophila is a sleep-like state', *Neuron*. (2000); 25: 129–38.

Prof Julian Huxley in The Beacon, for January 1922: 'M Coué has given us results. It is for science to discover and understand the mechanism by which these results are obtained, and, by that comprehension, to make them a permanent part of the heritage of humanity.'

Orton J. L., Émile Coué – The Man and His Work (1935): p 114.

Lyamin O. I. et al., 'Fur seals suppress REM sleep for very long periods without subsequent rebound', *Current Biology* (2018); 28(12): R699–R701.

Noble, Lady: *M Coué and Auto-Suggestion* (1924).

Orton J. L.: 'The roadway to where he stayed was lined with limousines and perambulators, bath chairs and sick beds.' *Émile Coué – The Man and His Work* (1935): p107.

Siegel J.: 'Who sleeps?', *The Scientist* (2016): https://www.the-scientist.com/features/who-sleeps-33973

Speirs R: Interviews with author, February and May 2017.

Tamaki M. et al.,'Night watch in one brain hemisphere during sleep associated with the first-night effect in humans', *Curr. Biol.* (2016); 26(9): 1190–4.

Waters R. C., 'Psychological terms are so frequently banded about in drawing-rooms and over the dinner table, that one is perhaps justified in saying that during the last decade the mind has taken the place of the stomach as a topical dinner-table subject. The Freudians and their various Nonconformist off-shoots have mainly been responsible for this popularizing of the subject', *So Built We the Wall*; Oxford: Hall the Printer Ltd., Littlegate (1937): p 16.

Westphal C. and Laxenaire M., Émile Coué: Amuseur ou précurseur? Émile Coué: Entertainer or Forerunner, *Annales Médico-Psychologiques, Revue Psychiatrique* (2012); 170(1): 38.

Yankauer, 'The Therapeutic Mantra of Émile Coué', *Perspectives in Biology and Medicine* (1999); 42(4): 489.

Yeates L. B., 'Émile Coué and his method (I): The Chemist of Thought and Human Action', *Australian Journal of Clinical Hypnotherapy & Hypnosis* (2016); 38(1): 3–27.

Acknowledgements

To Richard Waters, aka my great-great Uncle Dick: I feel indebted to my Uncle Dick and the memories I have of him, because if it wasn't for his work with Émile Coué and his passion for his own method, with all their books gathered on my shelves as a result, I would never have explored sleep from this starting point, and would likely never have fixed my chronic insomnia.

To Curtis Brown and Little, Brown: I would like to thank my agent Cathryn Summerhayes at Curtis Brown for her confidence in *Teach Yourself to Sleep* and for making it happen. And I'd like to thank my editor Zoe Bohm for seeing potential in this book and for her enthusiasm and insightful editorial suggestions, and Jillian Stewart and Jan Cutler for their meticulous line-by-line checks. I really appreciate the energy and hard work put in by the wider team at Little, Brown, in getting this book ready to go out into the world.

To the medics, scientists and experts: I am so grateful to those I interviewed, for their generosity in sharing their time and knowledge. I was thrilled to first discover Professor Peter Whorwell, given that his department is working with a 21st-century version of Richard Waters' method. He not only welcomed me into his hospital department on more than one occasion to discuss the benefits and workings of clinical hypnosis, but also invited me to sit in on his patient consultations, which was a fascinating experience. Dr Syed Shariq Hasan was equally generous, suggesting that I try clinical hypnosis first-hand, and he was so kind to provide a sleep script exclusively for *Teach Yourself to Sleep*.

I would also like to thank in the order that they appear on the page: Dr Laurence Sugarman, Executive Mind Coach and Cognitive Hypnotherapist, Kirsty Macdonald, who also wrote a sleep script exclusively for this book, Dr George Brainard, Dr Kyle S. Smith, Dr Tim Lomas, Professor Alison Wood Brooks, Professor Robin Dunbar, Dr Eugene Chang, nutritionist Samantha Perkins and Dr Mary Jane Minkin. All such great minds with an awe-inspiring amount of knowledge and expertise, and who it was a real pleasure to talk to.

To the librarians at the British Library: The British Library was a real home from home, but without the distractions, while I was researching and writing this book. A tranquil space where pretty much any book or journal I needed could be delivered to the section of the library that became my habitual hangout. And on those days when I couldn't work out how to access what I was after, the librarians would delve deep into the labyrinthian archives, to unearth them for me, which always felt like priceless treasure discovered at the end of a hunt.

To friends and family: So many friends and family members have given help, or cheered me on, along the way, and I am grateful to all of them. In particular, I'd like to thank Sarah Wasley for her belief in this book and for all the practical advice she gave, which helped propel me forward; also Lesley Thorne and Ruth Gavin for their valuable feedback, and Damian O'Hara for his photographic production.

I'm grateful to Cheryl McChesney and Gareth Jones for being there every step of the way, with urban forest walks and talks, advice and uplifting company, and Cecily Gatacre and Louise Stacey for their endless words of encouragement, their reader feedback on early drafts and the writer hideouts they created when solitude and head space was most needed.

Special thanks must go to my husband Chris Metzler, for doing everything he could to support me from day one. Also my mother, Rosemary Speirs, for first suggesting that I might want to write something about Coué (before I came across Waters' section on insomnia), and for telling me Waters' life story; and my children Kara, Blake and Dillon for their patience and for turning down the volume when I write at home.

To the reader: And I'd like to thank you, too, for reading this book.

Index